Life Before Birth

and

A Time To Be Born

Life Before Birth

and

A Time To Be Born

Peter W. Nathanielsz, M.D., Ph.D.

Foreword by Sir Graham (Mont) Liggins
Illustrations by Paula DiSanto Bensadoun

PROMETHEAN PRESS
ITHACA, NEW YORK
1992

ISBN: 0-916859-55-X

PROMETHEAN PRESS
P.O. Box 6827
Ithaca, NY 14851
U.S.A.

Prenatal care is a cooperation between you and your doctor. The information given here is correct to the best of my knowledge in GENERAL terms, but the ultimate responsibility for you and your pregnancy lies with yourself, your partner and your physician. Everyone is unique. P.W.N.

LIBRARY OF CONGRESS
Library of Congress Cataloging-in-Publication Data

Nathanielsz, P. W.
    Life before birth and a time to be born / Peter W. Nathanielsz ;
foreword by Sir Graham (Mont) Liggins ; illustrations by Paula
DiSanto Bensadoun.
        p.   cm.
    Includes index.
    ISBN 0-916859-55-X
    1. Fetus—Physiology.   2. Fetus—Growth.   3. Parturition.
I. Title.
RG610.N38   1992
612.6'4—dc20   92-26052
                                                                      CIP

PRINTED IN THE UNITED STATES OF AMERICA
97 96 95 94 93 92 5 4 3 2 1

This book is dedicated

*To my mother who shared my own life
before birth and taught me that you
should always aim to do your best; and*

*To my father who picked up a brown
paper bag containing a physically
handicapped baby on the steps of
Government House in Colombo, Sri Lanka
(at that time named Ceylon), and
decided to found the Ceylon Crippled
Children's Association.*

CONTENTS

FOREWORD

To those of average curiosity about the wonders of nature, it is likely that two great mysteries have stirred the imagination; and each concerns a birth. Who has not gazed into the heavens on a starlit night and wondered about the birth of the universe. And who hasn't been stimulated by the sight of a newly born baby to marvel at the unseen events within the mother's uterus that have led to the birth of such a perfect creation. But whereas one can readily obtain superb books (such as Stephen Hawking's *A Brief History of Time*) that provide a detailed account of modern cosmology written for lay persons but without skirting the complexities, scientists investigating fetal life have been remiss in failing to translate their science into terms that allow the public to fully share in the excitement of recent discoveries about life before birth. Much of what is written in this area is out of date, superficial and often an insult to the intelligence of the reader. Professor Nathanielsz now redresses the balance in a state-of-the-art book that contains most of the knowledge that I, as a fetal physiologist, carry in my head, written in a language that can be readily assimilated by readers unfamiliar with scientific jargon.

The author's credentials could not be bettered. Peter Nathanielsz was amongst the handful of pioneers who assisted at the birth about thirty years ago of the new discipline of fetology and he has remained at the forefront of what is now an enormous field. His laboratory has contributed many of the technical advances that now allow the most intimate details of fetal life to be examined with a precision equal to that of the cosmologists' radio-telescope.

If you are interested in knowing whether the fetus or the mother determines the time of birth, whether the fetus is asleep or awake, how one fertilized egg-cell can develop into a complete individual like—yet unlike—the parents, what goes on in the fetal brain, whether the fetus can tell the time or how the parents' lifestyle can harm the fetus, read this book. If any of those questions raises a spark of curiosity, read on but do not expect to consume the whole book in a single sitting for it is packed with fascinating descriptions of fetal systems and solid facts. This book will keep the reader occupied through much of the duration of fetal life and supplement parents' general prenatal education. Not that the book should be considered suitable for parents only—it is eminently suited to the needs of biology students, nurses, medical students and even obstetricians who want a comprehensive update on fetal physiology in a well-digested form.

It is little wonder that the secrets of fetal life have remained so secure until very recently despite curiosity and speculation dating back to Hippocrates and probably beyond. The arrival of the hi-tech age with its ultrasonic methods of visualizing the interior of human fetuses and its electronic methods of continuously observing every conceivable function in fetuses of animals had to be awaited before the private intrauterine world could be entered. Now it is routine for parents to watch their baby "breathing," urinating, thumb-sucking or whatever activity happens to coincide with an ultrasound scan and for scientists to safely measure such things as blood flow in the brain and umbilical cord or the size of the lungs and kidneys.

The idea that the fetus is just a miniaturized infant or adult is true to the extent that the fetal physiologist must be able to apply knowledge of every system obtained in adults, yet quite untrue in failing to recognize the many ways in which life before birth differs fundamentally from life after birth. For example, the fetus is weightless in her/his watery home and the environment is closer to that of an astronaut than to an earthbound individual. Many other instances of the uniqueness of the intrauterine environment emerge from the pages that follow, but I will reluctantly resist the temptation to reveal any more of the pearls that reward the reader in every chapter.

In these days when legislation, litigants and pressure groups have made it so important that our society is well-informed about science, I am delighted to have this opportunity to be the first to congratulate Peter Nathanielsz on producing what must surely remain the definitive Guidebook to the Intrauterine World.

Professor Sir Graham (Mont) Liggins, F.R.S., M.D.
Auckland, New Zealand
July 1992

PREFACE

The Child is the Father (Mother) of the Man (Woman)

William Wordsworth, *My Heart Leaps Up*

Until very recently the fetus was thought to be a passenger in the uterus, simply waiting for the great day the mother would give the signal, and her uterus would begin to contract and propel her baby into the world. We now know that far from being a passive participant in the birth process, the fetus is very much in command. The mechanisms which dictate the timing of normal birth are controlled by the brain of the fetus. In the last weeks of pregnancy the fetus makes his or her own responses to the challenges that could jeopardize optimal brain and body growth.

It is my hope that this book will serve as an introduction to the fascinating story of how we develop according to the blueprint laid down in our genes. This blueprint is used to control the exciting capabilities that the fetus possesses. This book focuses on fetal development in the last third of pregnancy; the breathing movements made by the fetus; the importance of functions carried out for the fetus by the placenta; the development of the fetal brain and the normal rhythms of fetal life; how the senses develop; how the fetus eventually gives the signal for birth; how the newborn adapts to the world outside the uterus; and other preparations the mother and fetus make toward a successful birth.

The major advances in our knowledge about life before birth have come from the application of many new approaches and a multitude of scientific disciplines. New biochemical techniques have allowed the measurement of hormones and other constituents in minute quantities of blood of both the mother and the fetus. Technological advances have enabled researchers to see inside the uterus using ultrasound. Today, many parents have video films of their children in the womb, moving their limbs and exercising their breathing muscles. Computers have enabled the storage and analysis of large amounts of data on fetal breathing movements, fetal brain waves, fetal heart rates and uterine contractility patterns. The techniques of molecular biology are providing information on the mechanisms cells use to divide and talk to each other. As we learn more about life before birth we will be able to help the next generation to prepare better for the challenges awaiting them.

The thanks of all the research community—and the community at large—should go to the National Institutes of Health, in particular the National Institute of Child Health and Human Development (NICHD), for their support of much of the research described in this book that is directed toward improving the chances of each newborn baby. I offer this book as a partial record to society of what has been achieved in improving our knowledge of normal development before birth, as well as normal and abnormal labor. Many independent foundations have also made significant contributions to research in this area. I would like in particular to thank the Lalor Foundation for several grants throughout my own research career. Often a small amount of financial support at a key moment in a research program can make all the difference. There are several donors, individuals and corporate, who have graciously supported the work at Cornell University of The Laboratory for Pregnancy and Newborn Research. I cannot name them here, but I am deeply indebted to them for their encouragement.

Each newborn child will only reach their full potential if the months of development in the uterus are free from adverse influences, providing the best possible environment for the baby. Premature birth occurs in about ten percent of births in the United States, and is linked to seventy-five percent of early infant deaths. Fifty percent of premature babies are likely to sustain long-term disabilities. More research is required if we are to conquer such problems as premature birth, fetal and newborn brain damage, sudden infant death syndrome, and intrauterine growth retardation. As in the past, only through basic scientific research will major breakthroughs occur. Today's advances were only made possible because of the research findings in previous years. We should not forget that in the same way today's research is tomorrow's benefit. This book provides some of the information society needs to evaluate the advances made in the knowledge that has led to the improvement of prenatal care that has been enabled by the NICHD and other funding agencies. I hope I have managed to transmit the wonder and awe that reaches me each day as I try to understand the intricacies of life before birth and a time to be born.

The more we understand about life before birth the sooner we will have the knowledge to provide the at-risk fetus with a *better* life before birth; and the sooner we will enable the fetus at risk of premature birth to choose a *better* time to be born.

Peter W. Nathanielsz, M.D., Ph.D.
Ithaca, New York
July 1992

ACKNOWLEDGEMENTS

This book is the product of thirty years of research into the mysteries of fetal development. It could not have been written without the intellectual stimulation of many colleagues and friends, a list too long to present here in full. I have had many great teachers to whom I owe an immense debt. I would like to thank especially Norman Rees who, in my high school years, taught me to marvel at the mysteries of life; W.C.W. (Bill) Nixon, who taught me the importance of obstetrics in relation to society; Richard Beard, who has been my mentor in obstetric research; and to Sir Graham (Mont) Liggins, who guided me in asking research questions and then assembling the techniques to answer them.

I am deeply indebted to my colleagues and students who have shown me the value of critical judgement and reservation of decision. For the excitement that comes from new knowledge and the pleasure of the day-to-day conduct of research I owe a immense debt of gratitude especially to Thomas McDonald, Barbera Honnebier, Jorge Figueroa, Dean and Tami Myers, Kenneth Lowe, John Buster, Patricia Jack, Richard Hardy, C.A.M. (Kees) Jansen, Peter Gluckman, Richard Harding, Robin Poore, Richard Weitzman, Maria Seron-Ferré, Murray Mitchell, Angela Massman, Molly Towell, Zbigniew Binienda, Thomas Reimers, Richard Wentworth, Gloria Hoffman, Barry Block, Don Schlafer, James Owiny, Mark Morgan, Susan Jenkins, Robin Gleed, Joshua Copel, Drew Sadowsky, Xiu Ying Ding, Luce Guanzini and many others. I am also grateful to my secretaries Karen Moore and Susan Shell for their unstinting help over the last ten years at Cornell University.

In William Shakespeare's great play, *Hamlet,* the elderly Polonius advises his son Laertes "The friends thou hast, and their adoption tried, Grapple them to thy soul with hoops of steel." Never were words more appropriate than for my life-long friend, Robert Lloyd, who read my manuscript more than once. His encouragement in the inevitable times of doubt was indispensable. I consider myself fortunate that one who is at the pinnacle of his busy artistic career, should have given attention to the scribblings of a scientist.

ACKNOWLEDGEMENTS

Finally, for the daily support of my wife, Diana, who has born with me the years of research and the mental investment in the gestation of this book. I recognize in our children, Julie and David, the energy that charted their own ways through life before birth; they and their generation will have the task of carrying the work forward.

Peter W. Nathanielsz, M.D., Ph.D.

Chapter 1

THE CHALLENGES OF FETAL LIFE

*And surely we are all out of the computation of our age, and every
man is some months elder than he bethinks him; for we live, move,
have a being, and are subject to the actions of the elements, and the
malice of diseases, in that other World, the truest Microcosm, the
womb of Our Mother.*

Sir Thomas Browne, *Religio Medici*, 1642

Life before birth was, until recently, a complete mystery. How we
develop in the womb was a riddle, the subject of speculation and
guesswork and shrouded in superstition. Research in the last thirty
years, using the powerful methods of modern biomedical technology, has helped reveal the amazing capabilities of the fetus in
the last three months or so before birth. We now know that the
fetus develops according to a finely tuned program. Life before
birth progresses precisely and deliberately from one stage to the
next according to a clear plan. In the last three months of his life in
the womb, the fetus develops the ability to respond and react very
purposefully to all manner of challenges that he faces even in the
protected environment in which he lives—the uterus. Moreover, we
now know that when things progress normally the fetus is very
much in control as to what goes on in that "other world, the truest
microcosm, the womb."

Technology is moving so fast that we are already ceasing to be
surprised by it. Obstetricians, and even pregnant mothers and
fathers, now take for granted the ability to study the unborn baby
using the ultrasound machine. Yet, ultrasonography is little more
than two decades old. We are already in danger of losing our sense

1

of wonder at being able to see the fetus moving and breathing. Technology has made available electronic recording devices that can print out the changes in the heart rate of the fetus as he responds to the sounds of his parents' voices. The obstetrician can observe how strenuous exercise by the mother affects her fetus. We can even take a blood sample from the baby's umbilical cord to analyze his detailed genetic make-up. We can measure the oxygen in his blood to assess how he is progressing, with only the slightest disturbance of his own private world. With these powerful new technologies many previously unanswerable questions about this crucial period of our own and our children's lives can now be answered with firm knowledge.[1]

The most amazing aspect of this fascinating time of human life is that the mother and fetus, although locked in the most intimate of physical relationships, are at all times two separate people. They are genetically distinct organisms. Until about twenty-two weeks of life, the fetus is totally incapable of sustaining himself without support from his mother. Thus, although structurally separated from his mother, she is his life-support. To conveniently distinguish between them scientists and obstetricians generally refer to the fetus as *he* and to the mother as *she*. The gender distinction is convenient and also serves as a useful reminder of the separateness of the two beings. Obstetricians generally refer to the baby before birth as the fetus and after birth as the baby.

We can now take the firm, clear scientific evidence available to us, combine it with sound reasoning based on the known facts of how our bodies work outside the womb, and put together an exciting picture of how the fetus develops his capabilities. It is important to understand the relationship between the physiological challenges that the fetus has to deal with in the uterus and those that confront the newborn baby in the minutes, hours, and days immediately after birth. In the womb, or uterus, the fetus has to develop systems for a life he has never experienced. The outside world is vastly different from the snug comfort of the uterus. The information to make appropriate responses correctly is locked in his genes. His predecessors, you and I, successfully rose to this challenge of being born, and fortunately we kept the blueprints of

---

[1] For an exciting description of the clinical uses of these techniques see *The Baby Doctors* by Gina Kolata, Dell Publishing Co., 1990.

how we did it in our genes. Consequently, we were able to pass the instructions on.

Using the outline plan provided in his genes, the developing fetus must respond to a multitude of changes imposed by his mother's activities. The food she eats, the exercise she takes, her alcohol and nicotine intake, and many other health hazards that come with her lifestyle all pose challenges over which he has no control but against which he must protect himself and make appropriate responses.

Assuming that his mother's lifestyle is not too self-destructive, however, the fetus uses her as a reservoir of nourishment and a secure environment while he sets about the momentous task of growing a heart, lungs, kidneys, digestive system, limbs, even fingernails, and most important of all, a brain. Everything has to be ready by the time of his birth when he makes the greatest transition he will ever be called upon to make. The sudden change from being a fetus, totally dependent on his mother, to a lifestyle as an independent newborn baby takes only a few minutes. The transition is violent, dramatic, rapid, and intense—a most awe-inspiring event. Given proper preparation, birth is a safe and normal event, and each individual birth is truly a great miracle.

The biggest single challenge to the fetus at the moment of birth is to break free of his dependence on the placenta, which has been his life-line for nine months. He has to accept responsibility for his own oxygen supply. Suddenly he has to be able to breathe air in and out of his lungs. How, you might ask, does he know how to breathe?

Throughout the whole of pregnancy his fetal lungs were collapsed. He received his oxygen directly into his blood supply through his placenta. His lungs were filled with only a small quantity of liquid. Within minutes of being born the baby must expand his lungs, get rid of the fluid, take in air, and let out the carbon dioxide. Everyone longs to hear the baby's first cry announcing that he made it, but not too many stop to think just what a challenging process the baby has just been through.

At the moment of fertilization, what we tend to call conception, the fetus is only a single cell containing genetic information from both his mother and father. This single cell produces two daughter cells, which then themselves divide. This process continues to form a multitude of cells. However, all the daughter cells are not the same. As they sort themselves out into groups to form the different organs of the fetal body, each daughter cell retains some characteristics and loses others. As if by magic, each cell knows its destiny. Some cells group together to form the muscle of the fetal heart, others become nerve cells. Scientists are just beginning to unravel the complex genetic and molecular codes that make sure that each organ develops "just right."

As well as dividing to form the various parts of the fetus, some of the cells make up the placenta and the membranes that form a sack around the fetus to protect and isolate him. The placenta also contains cells derived from the mother, making it a joint effort.

The fetus is not alone in changing and maturing. From very early on in pregnancy, the mother very rapidly notices new demands placed on her body. She notices the new ways in which her body is working. Her heart has to pump large amounts of blood through the placenta. She re-adjusts her food intake. She has to provide the building blocks for the fetus and placenta as well as the fuel they burn to stay alive. She needs extra energy to carry around the extra weight of pregnancy. Normally maternal blood pressure falls during pregnancy. A rise in the mother's blood pressure is abnormal and needs monitoring very carefully. It is certainly in the best interest of the fetus that his mother remain healthy and understand what is going on inside her. Mother and baby need to stay in tune with each other.

In the 1960s obstetricians made it much easier to know what was going on when they developed the ultrasound machine. It works rather like a video camera that can look into the uterus. Interestingly, the ultrasound was developed from instruments used during World War II for detecting submarines. Ultrasound waves pass easily through water and bounce back when they hit an object that is surrounded by water. The reflected soundwave is monitored by special detectors. Now the same technology is used to look at the fetus as he too lies surrounded by fluid.

From images produced using ultrasound we know that in the last weeks of pregnancy the developing fetus regularly and systematically exercises all the muscles he is going to need after birth. Of particular importance are the breathing movements that the fetus makes, exercising the muscles of his chest wall and diaphragm. In the last few weeks of fetal life, the fetus seems to undertake periodic bouts of breathing. Of course, there is no air for him to breathe as he is surrounded by fluid; he is only practicing.

Interestingly, however, if the fetus gets short of oxygen—for instance, if his mother smokes too much—then he stops breathing. This stoppage of breathing is called a paradoxical response to lack of oxygen. It is paradoxical because stopping breathing when he is short of oxygen is the exact opposite of what he will do once he is outside the uterus. Once outside the uterus, if he is short of breath he will breathe more deeply, like we all do while jogging or in high altitudes. The paradoxical response raises all manner of interesting issues.

The paradoxical response suggests, for example, that at the moment of birth the fetus/baby has to pull off a neat re-wiring of the circuits within his brain, reversing in a very short space of time what he has been doing during most of his fetal life. Now, as a newborn baby, he must breathe more vigorously when he needs more oxygen. Could it be that he sometimes gets confused? It would be only human. There is a line of thought that suggests that confusion about the appropriate response to lack of oxygen—a condition known as hypoxia—may be responsible for the mysterious and distressing Sudden Infant Death Syndrome (SIDS; also referred to as crib death). A baby with a blocked-up nose, or face down in a pillow, or in a stuffy room may get confused and revert to his old fetal habit of not breathing when he is short of oxygen. This theory has not been proven by medical science, but it is an example of the way painstaking researches into the changes that occur around the time of birth can produce important lines of enquiry in other fields. One never knows where research is going to lead.

The ancient Pharaohs of Egypt worshipped their placenta and it was carried before them on ceremonial occasions. It is certainly a unique organ. During the nine months of pregnancy the placenta acts as a fetal lung, digestive system, and kidney, and is a vital link to the energy-producing sources of the mother. Then suddenly at birth the fetus decides he doesn't want it anymore. The placenta is the body's only throw-away organ. It is fertile ground for scientific research. Scientists would like to know how it produces and secretes hormones, and because there are no nerve fibers going to the placenta, it is a mystery how the fetus signals to it. Recent research shows quite clearly that the fetus and placenta are sending messages back and forth, keeping up a continuous communication with each other to ensure that they work together toward the same goal. Scientists and obstetricians would like to know how the mother and fetus share responsibility for the placenta. For months during fetal life the fetus has to pump blood to the placenta and then at birth he finds he does not have to do that any more.

Surprisingly, adult structures are usually simpler than fetal structures. It is the target of the fetus to become an adult and once he gets there, physical life becomes simpler in many ways. En route, he has his own genetic program to help him find the way, but he has to have enough flexibility to cope with unexpected challenges as they arise from outside.

One important way the fetus differs from the adult is the complexity of the pathways along which he pumps his blood. The fetal bloodstream flows in a different pattern from that of the adult. The fetus only pumps a very small amount of blood to his lungs. To pick up oxygen, his blood must go to the placenta. The lungs are not the site of oxygen exchange in the fetus as they are in the adult.

In the fetus the quality of the blood that goes to his head and developing brain is very different from the quality of the blood that goes to his trunk and limbs. The blood supplying the fetal brain is better oxygenated than the blood that goes elsewhere. In adults the composition of the blood in the large arteries supplying all the regions of the body is the same, with the exception of that supplying the lungs. So at the time of birth a complete re-routing of the blood circulatory system takes place, and it all has to happen within minutes. There is no time for indecision. These changes are remarkable in their extent and rapidity. We are only now beginning to find clues as to how they take place.

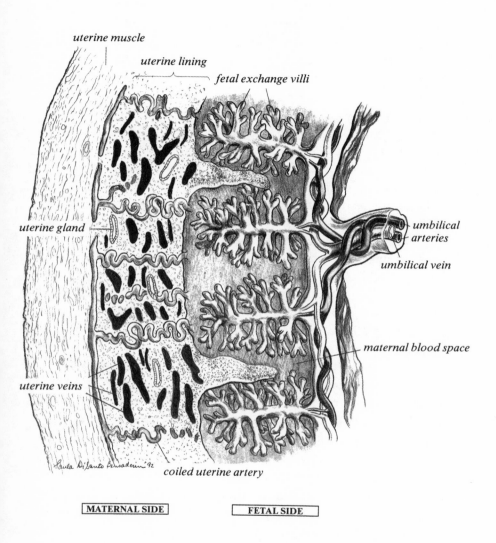

uterine muscle

uterine lining

fetal exchange villi

uterine gland

umbilical
arteries

umbilical vein

maternal blood space

uterine veins

coiled uterine artery

MATERNAL SIDE

FETAL SIDE

FIGURE 1.1
The placenta. A complex organ made up of a mixture of fetal and maternal cells.

Perhaps not surprisingly the fetus pumps his best blood to his brain. He knows instinctively that without a well-developed brain nothing else is going to work properly. Some of the most rewarding and potentially vital research being conducted by scientists today makes use of powerful modern technologies in a painstaking attempt to piece together how the brain develops. The 1990s have been declared the Decade of the Brain. One of the most intriguing frontiers of knowledge is the study of the development of the brain in the uterus.

What is already clear is that the fetal brain is always on the move, always working. For instance, there is something clearly visible on ultrasound that looks like rapid eye movement (REM), which is what we do when we dream. If the fetus is really dreaming, what on earth can he be dreaming about? The appearance of REM seems to suggest that he is aware of the outside world much more than one might think. Sounds, dietary changes, shocks, movement, and changes in light intensity are all examples of outside influences that might well provide him with plenty to dream about. Could it be true after all that Mozart learned his music in the womb and popped out ready to compose a symphony or two? Certainly there is much to suggest that what is going on in the mother's world deeply affects the behavior patterns of the fetus. If this is so, a great deal of a person's character and capabilities may be shaped in the womb along with all the mechanical bits of his body.

The fetus' prime concern is getting enough oxygenated blood to his brain. This is vital for normal brain development. The consequences of inadequate oxygen delivery to the brain can be long-term disability or brain damage. The fetus has developed ingenious mechanisms to maintain the oxygen supply to his brain by increasing brain blood flow when oxygen supply is poor. He keeps the blood and oxygen flowing to his brain at the expense of other parts of his body if necessary. This compensatory mechanism explains why the oxygen-deficient baby is often growth-retarded. He has retarded the rate of growth of his body in an attempt to protect his vulnerable developing brain. How the fetus tries to protect his brain at all costs, what the consequences are if these compensatory mechanisms fail, and how all this relates to such distressing conditions such as cerebral palsy, autism, and epilepsy are all important questions that modern technology is making it possible to tackle. What we are learning will one day help us to protect the fetus from the long-term consequences of episodes of oxygen lack. This knowledge will help reduce the incidence of brain damage and show us how to ensure that our children are born healthy.

Firm evidence exists to show that the twenty-four-hour day is one of the outside influences to which the fetus reacts in the uterus. There is now considerable interest in the scientific community in chronobiology. This is the science of biorhythms. Shift work is known to affect people's productivity. It is not just the traveling businessperson who worries about the effects of daily time shifts. The fetus can also show "jet lag in utero." He can also be affected by time and light; for instance, when daylight saving begins. It is obvious that some adults are so-called morning people and some are night owls. It could well be that these differences are learned in the womb. It is certainly true that there are twenty-four-hour rhythms for maternal and fetal heart rates. Both their heart rates are lowest at four in the morning and rise about twenty-five percent by ten in the morning. There is a prolonged and significant increase in the amount of time the fetus spends practicing his breathing between one and seven in the morning. We are not sure yet whether the fetus takes his cue from his mother for these heart and breathing rhythms or whether he controls them independently. We do know that the rhythms in concentrations of different hormones in the fetal blood are influenced by the concentrations of hormones in the maternal blood. It would seem that some fetal rhythms are self-imposed and some originate in the mother.

The importance of this line of enquiry is that by better understanding these rhythms and their function we can better provide for the needs of the newborn infant in his feeding and sleeping patterns. It is as a result of this work that dramatic changes are taking place in the management of the intensive care units for premature newborn babies. It is now accepted that the excessive hustle and bustle in these units is best avoided if at all possible.

Some babies are born undersize or growth-retarded, but this need not be a cause for alarm. Size is not everything. The newborn can catch up very quickly provided his brain has been properly nourished in the uterus. The real problem to worry about is not so much growth retardation before birth but brain retardation before birth. Fortunately, because of the high priority the fetus gives to his brain, it is usually remarkably well protected. To a large extent the fetus can control and pace his own development even when the provision of essential materials from the mother is disturbed or decreased. Quality of life, especially brain-life, is more important to the newborn than mere size.

With the knowledge of the importance of fetal brain development in mind, perhaps all pregnant women should be issued with T-shirts inscribed "Baby on Board—Don't Abuse." Pregnancy is not a time for smoking or drinking alcohol in anything more than the smallest amounts. Every mother should be aware that her lifestyle profoundly affects the development of her fetus. All the experimental and clinical studies conducted to date show how important abstinence—or at the very least, moderation—is when it comes to any form of drug-taking during pregnancy. We now have very firm information about the ways in which alcohol, tobacco, prescription drugs, and drugs of abuse can damage fetal development. The current cocaine and "crack" explosion is exacting a terrible toll. There is an enormous amount of research on the adverse effects of cocaine and other drugs on the fetal heart and brain. All the effects are bad. The studies show that the most harmful effects of cocaine are those that occur indirectly rather than the direct effects of cocaine crossing the placenta and intoxicating the fetus. Cocaine in the mother's blood can shut down the mother's blood supply to the uterus almost completely. This is potentially disastrous for the fetus. Cocaine does not need to cross the placenta to harm the fetus. The unborn baby is an astonishingly capable little creature but he cannot be expected to cope without oxygen. Voltaire had a very good point: "In ignorance, abstain." Your baby depends on you.

The traditional opinion of the mystery of birth was first precisely expressed over twenty-five hundred years ago by Hippocrates:

> *When the child is grown big and the mother cannot continue to provide him with enough nourishment, he becomes agitated, breaks through the membranes and incontinently passes out into the external world, free from any bonds. In the same way, among the beasts and savage animals, birth occurs at a time fixed for each species without overshooting it, for necessarily in each, nourishment will become inadequate. Those which have the least food for the fetus come quickest to birth, and vice versa. And that is all I have to say upon the subject.*

Until comparatively recently that was pretty much all that anyone had to say. In fact, any comments were essentially supposition heaped upon conjecture. Recent research, however, has completely changed the picture.

The most exciting finding is that birth, far from being the result of the mother's inadequacy or wish to get rid of her fetus, is a decisive act by the fetus. Because he is in charge, the fetus can align the correct program of development of his vital organs such as his brain and lungs with the timing of birth. The ability of the fetus to match his maturation to the duration of pregnancy is clearly of great value to the newborn in his need to adapt and respond to the challenges of life after birth. We now know which part of the brain contains the trigger mechanism for birth. As we shall see in Chapter 12, the fetus pulls the trigger many days before labor eventually occurs. The processes he sets off are very gradual, producing their final culmination in labor. Birth is not the sudden decision to be born that, on the surface, it appears to be. We should not ignore the role of the mother, but in determining the duration of pregnancy it appears that the fetus is the pilot and the mother the co-pilot.

If the fetus is a bit trigger-happy and fires the signal off too soon we may have a premature birth. The role of the fetus in determining the length of pregnancy is an extremely significant discovery because it paves the way for scientists and obstetricians to better understand the problem of prematurity. As we learn more and more about premature birth we are better able to prevent it, if necessary.

Prematurity is the major problem facing obstetricians. It is the great fear of many women. While overall only ten percent of babies are born prematurely in the United States, the incidence of prematurity varies greatly in different groups in society. This differential spread throughout society suggests that we need research from both medical and social scientists. As a result of extensive research, in the United States mostly supported by the National Institute of Child Health and Human Development, we are beginning to understand why prematurity occurs and learn how to tackle what is in fact a very serious problem. Although only one in ten babies is born prematurely, premature babies account for three quarters of birth-related deaths and half of all long-term neurological handicaps. Because the last twenty years has produced such outstanding advances in knowledge about life before birth it is now possible to dispel many fears. There have been great advances in the diagnosis and care of women in premature labor and our ability, aided by technology, to support the premature baby.

The neonatal intensive care unit can never be a complete replacement for the uterus, but the successes achieved by neonatologists in managing all but the very smallest premature babies are nothing short of miraculous. Isaac Newton, perhaps the greatest mathematician of all time, was born prematurely. It is said that he could have been placed in a pint pot. That says something for the amazing ability of the fetus to protect his brain against all odds. Neonatology, the modern study of the transition between fetal life and the immediate newborn period, would be impossible without the new scientific information on how the fetus matures.

Society desperately needs more information about normal and abnormal fetal development. The economic and social costs of managing premature babies and treating the consequences of prematurity are enormous. The annual conference of Governors of Southern States calculated that the cost of managing the problems posed by five premature babies equals the cost of providing adequate prenatal care for one hundred forty-nine women. Doctors in all fields of medicine are now thinking more often of prevention as an alternative to cure. In the field of premature birth, research into prevention would pay handsome dividends in terms of both cash savings and human happiness.

Passing the newborn baby into the arms of his parents signifies that a new and independent life has begun. The baby's body is struggling unseen with a whole host of new jobs he has to do. Now he has to get oxygen through his lungs, not the placenta; he has to learn to take his food through his digestive system and to cleanse his blood by evacuating waste through his kidneys; he has to control his own body temperature. If he's lucky he has caring parents to help him but when the chips are down, it's his life, his Great Adventure. Fortunately, he has taken time to prepare himself during life before birth.

The advances in understanding the miracle of life before birth and the birth process have done nothing to reduce the wonder of it. What all the complicated computerized machinery of modern biomedical research has revealed is that birth can be even safer and even more joyful with proper understanding and management. It is the purpose of this book to increase that understanding in the hope that we all may come to realize what responsibility we have for the shape of future generations.

Chapter 2

Egg Meets Sperm—What Happens Next

Nature's Rudiments and Attempts are involved in obscurity and deep night, and so perplexed with subtleties, that they delude the most piercing wit as well as the sharpest eye...In the reciprocal interchange of Generation and Corruption consists the Eternity and Duration of Mortal creatures. And as the Rising and Setting of the Sun, doth by continued revolutions complete and perfect time; so doth the alternative vicissitude of Individuums, by a constant repetition of the same species, perpetuate the continuance of ...[the species].

William Harvey, *Anatomical Exercitations Concerning the Generation of Living Creatures*, London, 1653, ex. XIV.

Ovulation is the release of the ovum (egg) from the ovary. It takes place about every twenty-eight days—a lunar month. The interval between ovulations varies slightly from woman to woman. Each ovum is contained within a grape-like cluster of cells called a follicle. In each monthly cycle, several follicles begin to mature and increase in size. One of these follicles (very occasionally two, or even three) becomes the dominant follicle. The dominant follicle is the follicle that will burst and release the ovum at ovulation. Occasionally more than one follicle will ovulate. Once in eighty occasions two eggs are ovulated, giving rise to a twin pregnancy; one in six and a half thousand times, three eggs are ovulated with the result that triplets will develop. Between the ages of fifteen and fifty a woman will ovulate about four hundred times.

As the dominant follicle develops, it pushes to the edge of the ovary and forms a bump on the surface. At ovulation the bump softens and eventually ruptures. The fluid in the follicle is released and with it the ovum surrounded by a sticky entourage of nutritive cells that will protect and nourish the ovum during the first few hours of its journey to the uterus. The egg's journey has begun.

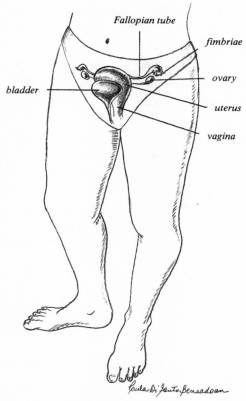

FIGURE 2.1
The female reproductive tract.

The Fallopian tube leads from the abdominal cavity into the uterus. At ovulation it plays an important role. The finger-like projections (fimbriae) around the opening of the Fallopian tube sweep backwards and forwards over the surface of the ovary positioning themselves to catch the ovum as it escapes from the surface of the ovary. It is likely that specific chemicals secreted by the mature follicle help to direct the fingers of the Fallopian tube to the exact site on the surface of the ovary at which the follicle will rupture and release the ovum. Even after release of the ovum, the follicle has an important role to play. Before ovulation, the predominant hormone produced by the follicle was estrogen. Now, as a result of new signals from the woman's pituitary gland, the follicle—now called a corpus luteum (literally "yellow body")— begins to secrete progesterone, a hormone that is vital to the maintenance of the pregnant state.

The environment within the Fallopian tube is ideally suited to nurture the ovum and the cells that surround it in their passage from the ovary to the cavity of the uterus. Fertilization takes place within the outer, wider part of the Fallopian tube. The time interval between ovulation and the deposition of sperm in the woman's reproductive tract at intercourse is not critical. The ovum can survive for twenty-four hours from the time of ovulation. If it is not fertilized in this period of time, the ovum will die. At intercourse, five hundred million sperm are ejaculated into the reproductive tract. Some of these may reach the Fallopian tube within an hour, others take their time. Because sperm are capable of surviving for five days in the Fallopian tube while still retaining the ability to fertilize the ovum, we see that the timing between intercourse and ovulation is not critical. Nature has an enormous investment in ensuring that the sperm and ovum are both in good shape when they meet, and has built several safety measures into the timing.

When the sperm find the ovum in the Fallopian tube, it is still surrounded by the nutritive cells that accompanied it from the follicle. These protective cells must be stripped away before a sperm can penetrate the outer casing of the ovum. Several hundred sperm finally reach the protected ovum. It is fortunate that there are so many sperm to work together in their task to free the ovum. The head-end of each sperm contains powerful enzyme proteins that rapidly dissolve the attachment of the surrounding cells away from the ovum. Once the surface of the ovum has been exposed, several sperm proceed to bore their way through its outer casing. A real race is now on. Millions of sperm originally started out on the quest but now just a few sperm compete for the ultimate prize. As soon as one sperm has succeeded in burrowing through to the ovum, a chemical reaction occurs within the ovum that prevents any other sperm from making it through. One sperm is enough for the final act of fusion of the male and female genetic information needed to create a new individual.

The genetic information that is handed down from generation to generation is contained in the genes. Genes are very large molecules that contain the detailed program, or blueprint, for all the activities of the cell. They are lined up on the chromosomes within the nucleus (control center) of each of the cells in the body. Each chromosome is like a necklace of pearls with each pearl representing a gene. There are forty-six chromosomes in the nucleus of each cell except the gametes, or sex cells. The ovum, the female gamete, contains only twenty-three chromosomes, half the number that are present in each of the other cells in the body of the mother-to-be. Similarly, each one of the millions of sperm, the male sex cells, contains only twenty-three chromosomes, again half the number present in each of the other cells in the father's body. This halving of the number of chromosomes in the sex cells is a necessary preparation for the fusion of genetic information from the mother and father that will be passed on to the next generation. The twenty-three male and twenty-three female sex chromosomes, when brought together at fertilization, give the resulting union a total of forty-six chromosomes, the same as in all other cell nuclei.

The cell is the basic building unit of the body. There are many small organisms that consist of just a single cell. The most commonly known is the little amoeba that slides along in ponds, putting out small blips as it makes its way, apparently gliding effortlessly over the surface with which it is in contact.

The ovum contains all the basic components of the cell. The whole cell is enveloped by a membrane called the plasma membrane. This membrane is made up of two layers of fat and protein molecules that act as a barrier between the cell and the fluid outside. This barrier enables the cell to control the passage of molecules into and out of the cell. The cell is thereby protected from changes in its environment. Inside the plasma membrane is a specialized thin porous jelly-like fluid through which molecules shuttle backwards and forwards performing their specific tasks. At the center of the cell is the command center, the nucleus, that contains the genetic code. At most times in the life of the cell the individual chromosomes cannot be seen. They are hidden within the nucleus. Just before the cell begins to divide, the chromosomes become apparent as small worm-like structures.

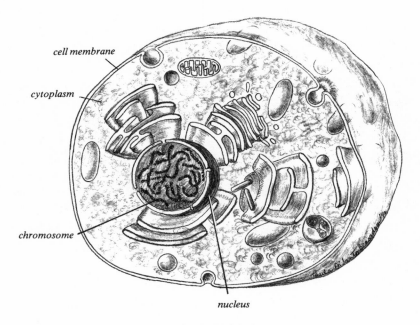

cell membrane

cytoplasm

chromosome

nucleus

FIGURE 2.2

Diagrammatic representation of the major components of the cell—the software program for development is contained within the nucleus on the chromosomes.

As we have seen, the ovum is fertilized by only one sperm. As a result of the fusion of a single sperm with the ovum, a single cell is produced that contains the correct number of chromosomes, forty-six for all the cells of the adult body. If a preliminary halving of the mother's and father's chromosomes had not taken place, the fertilized ovum, the first cell of the new organism, would contain ninety-two chromosomes, twice the amount of genetic information necessary for production of the new member of the species. The cells of individuals of the next generation would contain one hundred eighty-four, and so on, doubling with each generation. Clearly this doubling of instructional information contained within the genetic code would have impossible consequences for each new generation.

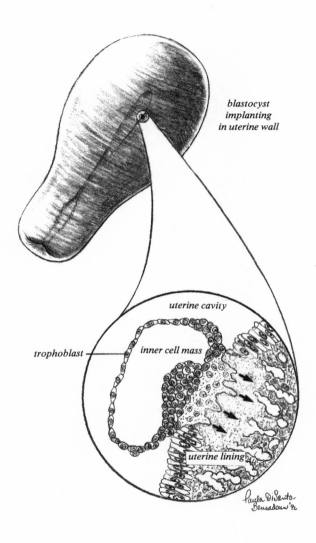

blastocyst implanting in uterine wall

uterine cavity

trophoblast

inner cell mass

uterine lining

FIGURE 2.3

A section through a blastocyst. The inner cell mass will give rise to the fetus; the trophoblast will give rise to the placenta and fetal membranes. The blastocyst is beginning to implant in the uterine wall.

In the early hours after fertilization, the genetic material of the mother and father comes together to form the zygote. Within twelve hours or so the first division of the zygote into two cells takes place. As the developing ball of embryonic cells is propelled slowly toward the uterus, division of cells continues to occur so that the cell number doubles about every twelve hours. At this stage there are many dangers that may prematurely cut short the continued development of the embryo. The folds within the Fallopian tube may contain scars from previous infections that may hold up the growing ball of cells. The ball of cells is called a morula, from the Latin word for a mulberry, which it resembles. Should the morula stick to the wall of the Fallopian tube and try to develop there, such a pregnancy is called an ectopic pregnancy, ectopic meaning "not in the right place." The Fallopian tube has much thinner walls than the cavity of the uterus and does not have the same large blood supply. Ectopic pregnancies eventually die and may often cause considerable trouble because the Fallopian tube may burst and create an emergency situation.

Three to four days after fertilization the morula has developed a fluid-filled cavity within it and is now called a blastocyst. At this stage the blastocyst enters the uterine cavity. Already we are beginning to see the differentiation of the individual cells, all derived from the initial zygote, into different types with different functions and fates. The outer wall of the blastocyst is called the trophoblast and this will develop into the placenta and the membranes that cover the fetus. Looking down a microscope at this stage we can make out a very important group of cells on the underside of one area of the trophoblast. This group of cells is called the inner cell mass. The inner cell mass cells will develop into the embryo, the fetus, and eventually the newborn baby.

At this stage the protective outer casing that was present around the ovum still surrounds the blastocyst, but it soon breaks down. This allows the developing blastocyst to come directly into contact with the lining of the uterine cavity. Well before the end of the second week of life, the blastocyst has embedded itself completely within the uterine wall.

It is through the microscope that the embryologist gets a close-up look at cells dividing, giving rise to more cells for the growing embryo. Although the individual cell can grow to some extent, cell growth is limited as the larger the size of the cell the greater the distances over which oxygen and other nutrients have to diffuse to get to all parts of the cell. The interchange of substances within the cell and the environment around it can only take place through the plasma membrane that encloses the cell. Because the volume increases faster than the surface area of the plasma membrane, there comes a point when the surface area is too small to sustain all the activities of the increased volume of the cell. At this point, or earlier, the cell must divide if growth is to continue. Cell division to produce larger numbers of cells is indispensable to major growth.

The single-cell zygote contains all the information codes it needs to form any one of the wide variety of different cells of the body. These information codes are very like software in a computer. They are stored in the genes on the chromosomes in the nucleus. Cell differentiation is the process by which each cell specializes, deciding to focus its activities on a selected few of the many functions for which it has the necessary internal program.

The human body can be likened to the complex society in which we live. A society that is composed of individuals with identical capabilities can only perform that set of tasks. The wider the variety of capabilities of the individuals, the more diverse will be the output of that society. So it is with the human body. To move around we need muscle cells. To feel objects close to us, to hear sounds and see sights at a distance we need sensory cells. To convey messages from the sensory cells to our central computer, the brain, and then from the brain to our muscle cells to move out of danger, or toward a desired goal, we need nerve cells. To digest the food we eat, we need gland cells in our digestive system. To store food in times of plenty against the possibility of times of food shortage we need fat cells. Each type of cell is an example of differentiation to perform critical roles in the life of the whole organism. The body needs a very wide variety of cell types to achieve the rich potential of human life. One might say that variety and tolerance of differences is equally necessary for the health of society, or as it is appropriately called, the body politic.

To some extent growth and differentiation are mutually exclusive. Once a cell has differentiated it does not usually grow any more. Rather it focuses its activities on performing the specialized function it has opted to undertake on behalf of all the other cells of the body. The most extreme example is the mature nerve cell, which has completely lost the ability to divide. At birth you and I had all the nerve cells that we will ever have. Fortunately, as we grow older we can learn to put them to ever more complex use, but we cannot increase their number. Unlike the nervous system, however, other tissues maintain a reservoir of primitive cells that can still divide when called upon to replace dying cells. A good example is the red blood cell. A reservoir of primitive cells (known as stem cells) is maintained in the bone marrow, liver, and other sites so that constantly each day as some red cells die, some of the reserve cells differentiate into mature red blood cells, escape into the blood, and carry oxygen around the body.

Another major technological advance was the development of methods to grow cells from embryos in culture and observe their differentiation. Nerve cells being cultured can put out finger-like extensions, which engage each other in conversation. Culture experiments can be combined with electrical stimulation of the cells to show that the conversations between cells can actually modify their development. If we grow two groups of nerve cells side by side in a dish and allow them to establish connections, we can alter the rate of formation and type of connection between cells in the two groups by electrically stimulating the cells in one group so that more messages pass to the other group of cells. This experiment has important implications. It shows how the richness, or otherwise, of the environment during all stages of development, both before as well as after birth, may influence the brain's development. The importance of outside stimulation should not be so surprising. Muscles grow if they are exercised; likewise the increased use of the connections between nerve cells (called synapses) influences the growth and development of the active cells.

Much of our understanding of how cells grow and divide has come from the study of plant and animal cells. The science of embryology owes a great debt to the study of the growth and differentiation of frogs' eggs. As a scruffy ten-year-old with knobbly knees below my short pants, I used to scoop out frogs' spawn in a net from puddles on a World War II bomb site. Observing the growth and differentiation of the jelly-like frogs' spawn into tadpoles and the subsequent differentiation of the tadpoles into mature frogs was a period of sheer wonder for me. "How," I would ask myself, "does the tail know when to fall off?" and "What governs the appearance of the legs on the sides of the torpedo-shaped tadpole?" That was 1951. I did not know then that at Cambridge University, only sixty miles north of where I was scooping up the brackish water from the bomb craters, Francis Crick and James Watson and their colleagues were about to show how the cell stores the computer program that accomplishes the task of guiding and controlling cellular differentiation. The new methods of molecular biology would revolutionize our thinking about the hardware and software in the cell's computer.

The molecular make-up of the genetic code has been the subject of intense research in the last decade and the amount of information gathered appears overwhelming. Governments throughout the world have joined together to begin creating a map of the structure of all the genes and their relationship to each other on the chromosomes. This project, called the Human Genome Project, is a multi-billion dollar undertaking, which draws together the work of many molecular biologists. The goal is to complete this fundamental compilation of the blueprint of the human body in the next decade. As time passes, this vast amount of detail will be assimilated into fundamental basic concepts, including how the fetus develops in the uterus.

The abundance of information now available is in stark contrast to the knowledge base available over the preceding two thousand years. Nevertheless, Aristotle stumbled on the right idea when he guessed that the embryo developed from maternal and paternal components. However, subsequent medical philosophers lost their way and reasoned that the next baby exists preformed in the unfertilized egg. They ignored the problem of a contribution from both mother and father to the next generation. They also ignored the philosophical need to explain where the seeds of the third, fourth, fifth, and subsequent generations are located. If the unfertilized egg contains the next generation, perfectly preformed within it, then the generation after that must also be present in the egg and so on *ad infinitum*. This idea reminds me of the Russian metreshka, or nesting doll, that contains another doll fitted inside her. Remove both metreshkas and one usually finds another identical metreshka within and so on. The most significant feature about metreshkas is that they are often identical. People are not.

The infinitely-small-metreshka theory has two major flaws. First, the atomic theory of matter states that we can only split compounds down into their constituent atoms—after that we either have to stop, or split the atom. So, when do we get to the last metreshka? Even more important, the infinitely-small-metreshka concept does not allow both parents a role in contributing to the make-up of their offspring. Modern genetics has clearly shown us how the combination of different characteristics from mother and father eventually give rise to unique individuals similar in some ways to their parents but nevertheless with unique abilities.

I am reminded of the story in the first chapter of Stephen Hawking's magnificent book on the origin of the universe. An impossibility similar to the infinitely-small-metreshka theory is discussed. The impossible concept is that of the ancient opinion that the universe sits atop a tortoise. In the story, as Hawking tells it, a well-known scientist once gave a public lecture on astronomy. He described how the earth orbits around the sun and how the sun, in turn, orbits around the center of a vast collection of stars called our galaxy. At the end of the lecture a little old lady got up and said "What you have told us is rubbish. The world is really a flat plate supported on the back of a giant tortoise." The scientist gave a superior smile before replying "What is the tortoise standing on?" "You're very clever young man, very clever," said the old lady "But it's turtles all the way down!"[1]

Similarly, the concept of infinitely small metreshkas within infinitely smaller metreshkas is an untenable explanation for the mechanisms used to pass on the program of life from generation to generation.

---

[1] *A Brief History of Time: From the Big Bang to Black Holes*, Stephen Hawking, 1988, Bantam Books.

The turning back of erroneous ideas requires courage to stand up against the "correct" ideas of the day. Understanding can only advance when we approach the data we have without preconceived notions. Columbus was told the world was flat; Lord Kelvin, the Nobel Prize winning physicist, said that "heavier-than-air flying machines are impossible." Many excellent examples of the true scientific prophets who had the courage to buck the system of current scientifically correct thought are given in Julius Comroe's excellent book the *Retrospectroscope*.[2] The "retrospectroscope" is an instrument of the mind. Those who do not wish to repeat history should cherish and develop their own retrospectroscope.

The science of embryology has made astonishing strides in recent years with ever closer examination of the detailed structure of cells. New findings constantly amaze us as they reveal the magic of the process. Experimental observations constantly challenge assumptions bred of half-thought and prejudice and constantly open up new targets for yet more research in the ceaseless search for clearer, more precise, understanding.

The knowledge, for instance, that when the egg meets the sperm the resulting cell contains all the genetic information necessary to set in motion a process that will result in a unique human being, is knowledge that challenges many traditional philosophies, religions, and folklore. We shall see that the expression of this unique capability of the egg and sperm is dependent on environmental conditions within the uterus and interactions with the maternal organism. Thus, some may consider that the individual capacities of the sperm and unfertilized egg constitute life just as much as the fertilized egg. We also know that the fertilized egg has many developmental hurdles to jump before it becomes a viable fetus.

The intellectual and philosophical repercussions of this knowledge have still to be properly absorbed and digested. Our moral philosophy has yet to evolve a system of thought that fully accepts man's physical being as a product of a relentless and predictable process of cell growth and differentiation.

---

[2] *Retrospectroscope*, Julius H. Comroe, Jr., 1978, Von Gehr Press (sole distributor Perinatology Press, Ithaca, N.Y.).

Chapter 3

TASKS FOR FETAL ORGANS

For thou has possessed my reins: thou hast covered me in my
mother's womb. I will praise thee; for I am fearfully and wonderfully
made...

Psalm 139

The closely packed cluster of cells that make up the developing morula are not all equal. One small group of cells soon sets itself apart. These cells are called the inner cell mass, a disc of cells, initially a layer just a single cell thick. The inner cell mass will eventually give rise to all the cells that comprise every organ in the fetus. There is a long way to go; many divisions and much diversification must occur. Initially the inner cell mass divides to form three distinct layers beneath the outer casing of the spherical blastocyst. These three layers are called the ectoderm (or outer layer), mesoderm (or middle layer), and endoderm (or inner layer). Each layer develops into different tissues. Biologists define a tissue as a group of similar cells gathered together in one place, ready to perform one or more specific functions on behalf of the whole body.

By the end of the second week after fertilization a small bubble appears in the inner cell mass disc, separating these cells from the outer trophoblast. This bubble is filled with fluid. It grows to form what is called the amniotic cavity. The amniotic cavity continues to enlarge throughout the first weeks of pregnancy until it completely surrounds the fetus. The fluid in the amniotic cavity is colloquially called the "waters." This fluid is released at the time of birth.

At the same time a clearly defined column of cells grows forward along the eventual midline of the embryo. This column of cells, called the notochord, is the first indication of the future vertebrae of the spinal column. Notochord cells issue instructions that result in the differentiation of other tissues, especially the brain and spinal cord. By the end of the second week the embryo has a clear orientation of front and back, right and left, and head and tail ends.

During the third week after fertilization the ectoderm above the notochord thickens to form a tube that represents the beginnings of the spinal cord. These fundamental phases of development of the nervous system in the third week explain why the embryo is particularly sensitive at this critical stage of development to toxic substances that can adversely affect development of the brain. At this stage the primitive cells of the embryo have not committed themselves to their individual final tasks. If anything prompts them to make an incorrect decision, major and irreversible malformations may occur. In Chapter 12 we will see how a dramatic example of a malformation of the fetal brain results if the pregnant sheep eats a particular toxic plant, a type of skunk cabbage, on the fourteenth day of her pregnancy. The abnormal development of the fetal brain results from one specific toxic compound in the skunk cabbage. Although this malformation occurs at an early stage of pregnancy it eventually results in prolongation of the pregnancy past the time that normal delivery should have occurred. There are many other examples that could be quoted in humans and animals to show that the developing brain is particularly vulnerable to damage at this early stage of embryonic life.

Recent advances in our detailed understanding of how individual molecules interact within and between cells are beginning to define the mechanisms responsible for all this purposeful movement of cells from one location to another. For example, we now know the chemical nature of some of the messages that cells send to each other when they wish to get together in specific groups.

By the end of the third week the embryo has undergone segmentation, rather like an earthworm, and now consists of zones like stacked circular tires. Each segment will give rise to a different part of the body's long axis. The repetition of structures in segments is best seen in the chest. There, each vertebra and the attached rib is produced from one embryonic segment. By the end of the third week the primitive digestive structures are beginning to form.

A major feature of embryonic and fetal development is the common occurrence of death of cells. Almost from the very start of fetal life, some cells are programmed for a specific function at a critical period of development. After this task is accomplished they die. Cell death is a major feature of the way embryonic tissues and organs develop. These short-lived, yet important, cells seem to function on the basis of Andy Warhol's statement that "In the future, everyone will be famous for fifteen minutes." They perform their role in a brief span of time and are gone, leaving no progeny to carry on their work. Their instructions, like those for all cells, however, are preserved for the next generation in the genetic code of the cells that live on.

With the help of these disposable cells, the fetus develops some special organs that are specifically adapted to the unique environment he experiences in the uterus, and that will be of no use to him in the outside world after birth. The most obvious of these disposable organs are the placenta and the membranous sac that surrounds the fetus.

The placenta is the joint fetal and maternal organ that enables the maternal and fetal blood systems to come extremely close to each other without directly mingling. It is the component that makes it possible for two entirely separate organisms to live in such close proximity.

During the first four weeks of its existence the embryo makes the construction of the placenta its top priority. It is to be the fetal life-line for the next eight months. The embryo sets to work on shaping the placenta from the second week after conception. The outer layer of the embryo has great invasive powers and nudges its way into the lining of the mother's uterus. By the end of the second week of life the embryo is completely buried within the uterine wall. During this second week the embryo burrows further and further into the lining of the uterus and he begins to break into his mother's blood capillaries. As a result maternal blood forms little pools. Columns of trophoblast cells and the fetal blood vessels inside them form finger-like projections (called villi) which dip into the pools of maternal blood. Oxygen in the maternal pools of blood has only to traverse a relatively short distance to get into the fetal blood. The fetus is on his way to ensuring that he has close access to his mother's blood system. As yet, however, fetal blood is not flowing from the fetal cells that line these pools of maternal blood to the distant tissues of the fetus. He must develop some of his own blood vessels quickly. The blood in the maternal pools of the placenta is drained back into the maternal circulation. At no point are the maternal and fetal blood systems directly in contact. This remarkable separation of maternal and fetal blood is clearly seen when looking at the placenta down a microscope. The placenta provides an opportunity for the maternal and fetal blood to come extremely close to each other, but without direct intermingling.

At one edge of the developing embryonic disc a thickening of cells can be seen that connects the developing embryo to the trophoblast. This connecting stalk forms the umbilical cord. Umbilical arteries and veins form within the umbilical cord thereby connecting the developing fetal heart to the blood vessels in the placental villi. With the formation of the umbilical vessels oxygen and food will be whisked from what will be the placenta along the waterways of the blood system to the active fetal cells. The major steps in the development of the placenta are well under way by the fourth week.

Until the umbilical vessels are fully formed, oxygen and food can only get to the fetal cells by diffusion. Diffusion works as a gradual seepage of nutrients through the walls of each cell into the next. The slow nature of diffusion would limit the growth of the embryo to a sphere only one or two millimeters in radius. The evolution of the placenta is indispensable to the development of complex life forms that pass their early stages of development within their mother.

Obviously other organisms have the same problem during their development. The hen's egg is an excellent example. The hen provides a yolk sac for the chick so that there are enough nutrients available to provide all the energy and structural growth for the full

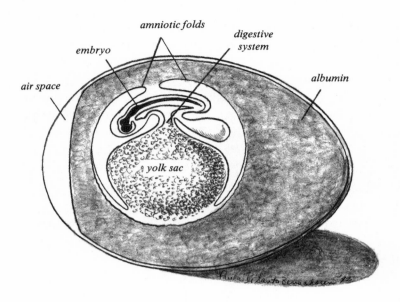

amniotic folds

embryo

digestive system

air space

albumin

yolk sac

FIGURE 3.1
Schematic diagram of the chick egg showing the air space within the shell.

twenty-one days of the chick's development. The chick gets oxygen in the egg across a thin membrane stretched across the egg next to a large air bubble called the air sac. The chicken's egg is permeable to gases so that oxygen can diffuse into the air sac and carbon dioxide can diffuse out. The egg is a remarkable self-contained package of life, comparatively simple in its mechanisms. Compared with the infinite complexity of the human, however, the chicken is a relatively simple creature.

The placenta in women is usually composed of a single disc. Occasionally the fetal vessels in two separate areas of the trophoblast may connect with the umbilical vessels in the umbilical cord. When this happens two placental discs are formed. When two discs are present, the umbilical cord is inserted into the larger disc and branches of the umbilical artery go from the primary to the secondary disc to supply it with fetal umbilical arterial blood. Branches of the umbilical vein drain back from the secondary disc to the main veins in the primary disc. The two-disc placenta only occurs in less than two percent of human pregnancies.

The placenta is thus a complex organ made up of both maternal and fetal tissues. The fetal component contains several distinctive types of cell, each type specialized to perform a different function. Major advances in our knowledge of placental function in the last twenty years have been possible because of three research approaches: first, the development of powerful microscopical techniques; second, the ability to culture or grow cells obtained from the placenta, and third, studies in animals on the factors that regulate the passage of oxygen and nutrients across the placenta. Later, we will look at these functions in greater detail.

The placenta may seem to be a peripheral, throw-away organ of only marginal impact on the normal growth and central development of the fetus. Nothing could be further from the truth. Correct placental function is absolutely crucial to the proper development of the fetus. The interrelationship between the cells of the placenta and the cells of the fetus is a fascinating example of how the multitude of cell types developed from the single fertilized egg work together. However, things can sometimes go wrong. In times of shortage, for example, the placenta and fetus can end up having to compete with each other. If placental function is inadequate for the fetus, growth retardation may occur. Critical aspects of fetal growth will be considered in detail in several chapters. In the next few years one of the goals of research in this area must be to develop methods to see how we can assist the placenta in its fundamental task of providing for the fetus in the best possible way.

For the first twenty weeks or so of life the fetus is protected by the amniotic cavity, which provides a cushion of fluid resembling a private swimming pool in which the fetus can develop. The amniotic cavity is surrounded by a membrane called the amnion, which is part of the fetal membranes. During this time the fetus is totally surrounded by amniotic fluid, which acts as a buffer. As we shall see later, after twenty weeks the amount of amniotic fluid is no longer adequate to completely surround the fetus and he comes into contact with the uterine wall at several points. Thus, he is affected by any squeezing that results from contraction of the uterus, which may have consequences that are of great importance to fetal development. The squeezes exerted on the fetus stimulate the fetus and result in changes in brain function as will be seen in the chapter on the fetal brain.

There is considerable folklore about the fetal membranes. In years gone by if the fetal membranes did not break during delivery it was considered a very lucky omen. An unbroken amnion, or caul, around the baby was supposed to predict that he would not die at sea! Such a prediction was of no little importance in seafaring communities. True or not, the fetal membranes are no longer considered the inert "wrapping paper" they were once thought to be. At the beginning of pregnancy the membranes press against the wall of the uterus and are an important means for nutrients to pass from the mother to the fetus before the formation of the placenta. The many active cells in the membranes produce a large number of very active biological compounds with many physiological functions. The products of the fetal membranes are well placed to play a role by carrying messages from the fetus to the mother, especially during the process of labor and delivery.

By the fourth week of life we can detect how the embryo is setting up the blood circulation system, which will serve to protect the development of his brain. The primitive fetal heart and vascular system can be seen as a single tube running in a head-to-tail direction. Local thickenings in the head end of the tube can be seen that will give rise to the heart, dividing it into an atrial portion toward the head end and a ventricular portion nearer the tail end. Both of these areas are again divided into two so that the four-chambered heart is formed. The division, or septum, between the right and left atria contains a hole with a flap on its left side that acts as a one-way valve allowing blood to pass from the right atrium to the left atrium. Blood does not pass in the reverse direction unless there is some abnormality of development.

Initially a single large vascular tube leads away from the heart. This single arterial trunk is split into two by the formation of a spiralling partition down its center. One half remains connected to the right ventricle and becomes the pulmonary artery, which feeds blood to the lungs; the other half is connected to the left ventricle and forms the aorta. The aorta is the major artery of the body. It arches forward toward the head end of the developing embryo, giving off the large arteries to the head and arms before turning to run along the spine toward the tail end to supply the developing abdominal and leg structures. The umbilical arteries that carry blood from the fetus to the placenta come off the aorta at its very end. A very important channel—the ductus arteriosus—connects the aorta and pulmonary arteries at a point after the arteries to the head have left the aorta. The importance of the ductus arteriosus is that it provides a connection between the right and left sides of the circulation, and allows blood to bypass the non-functional fetal lungs.

Arteries lead the blood away from the heart. They gradually break up into smaller and smaller tubes until the blood is in very thin capillaries. Oxygen and nutrients can diffuse through the thin wall of the capillaries into active fetal tissues. Thus, they provide the cells in the tissues with the materials they need for their energy production as well as the building materials needed for cell growth and division. To provide a pathway for blood to return to the heart, capillaries must join together to form small veins. The small veins flow into each other forming larger veins. Initially there are two large umbilical veins formed to return blood from the placenta to the fetus. During the fifth week one disappears. The remaining umbilical vein drains into the fetal inferior vena cava, the large vein that returns blood from the legs and abdomen to the heart. This blood from the placenta streams along in the inferior vena cava kept well separated from the other blood in this large vessel. As the inferior vena caval blood arrives at the right atrium, the well-oxygenated blood from the placenta is directed by a little bump in the wall of the right atrium across and through a small hole that exists in the wall that separates the right atrium from the left atrium. This hole is called the foramen ovale. The well-oxygenated blood goes directly to the brain. This ability to separate well-oxygenated blood and poorly oxygenated blood in the same vein (the inferior vena cava) is critical to the normal development of the fetal brain. The foramen ovale closes up immediately after birth.

The most important consequence of these developments in the primitive cardiovascular system is that the quality of blood going to the fetal brain is very different from that going to the tail end of the fetus and placenta. In times of need the fetus uses some very clever strategies to preserve supplies of oxygen and food for his developing brain, his most favored and important organ.

At birth the foramen ovale should close completely and permanently. If the flap covering the foramen ovale is too small to cover the hole, a permanent defect may remain between the right and left atria. This defect will allow blood to pass between the two atria, something that should not normally happen after birth. This deficiency in the wall between the atria, often called a "hole in the heart," may come in all sizes. Of course the larger the defect, the more blood will pass through after birth. Less commonly, a hole in the heart may occur between the two ventricles if the septum that grows between the two sides is not complete. These rare defects can now be seen during fetal life on the ultrasound, and surgeons are able to close them at the optimal time after birth.

The beginnings of the embryonic gut, or digestive tract, are also clear by the fourth week. The digestive tract is formed from both endoderm and mesoderm, two of the three layers of cells in the developing inner cell mass. The endoderm gives rise to the lining of the digestive system and the digestive glands, such as the pancreas, that bud off from the lining. The mesoderm gives rise to the muscle that propels food materials down the digestive system. During the fourth week of embryonic life the primitive digestive tract consists of a foregut, midgut, and hindgut. The foregut and hindgut develop so that they are in continuity with the amniotic cavity. Thus, the fetus is able to swallow amniotic fluid. Material from his pharynx can also pass in the other direction into the amniotic fluid. The fetus also passes feces into the amniotic fluid. These feces are called meconium and consist of the thick mucus from the digestive glands and the cells that slough off the digestive lining as it grows.

Several important structures grow out from the developing digestive tube. Knowing how they form can give strong clues to the nature of many abnormalities of development that may not show up until years after birth. For example, the thyroid gland grows out

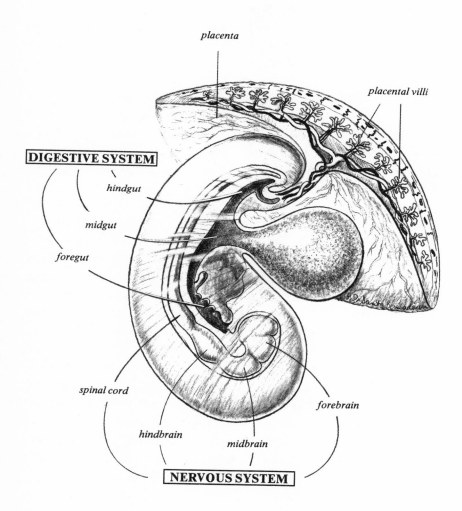

FIGURE 3.2

The developing human embryo and placenta. Villi from the fetal surface of the placenta dip down into a lake of maternal blood.

from a little pouch in the floor of the mouth, growing downward until it comes to rest at its final destination in the neck. On rare occasions small pieces of thyroid gland may be left behind along the track. If for any reason the thyroid becomes over-stimulated, for example, because the mother, and thus the fetus, becomes short of iodide, small thyroid overgrowths may form along the track.

The beginnings of many organ systems are distinguishable for the first time during the fourth week of embryonic life. At this time a pouch appears in the foregut just behind the developing pharynx. This pouch is called the laryngo-tracheal diverticulum because it will form into the larynx, trachea, and lungs. The laryngo-tracheal diverticulum develops rapidly to form the trachea and then divides to form the right and left lungs. The division continues, each branch getting smaller and smaller, until at last the small air sacs are formed within the lungs. It is across the thin membranes lining these air sacs that gases will be exchanged with the external environment after the baby is born. The pulmonary blood vessels, that is, the blood vessels of the lungs, divide into small capillaries that pass over the surface of the air sacs to enable the blood to come into close proximity with the air within the cavities. It should be remembered, however, that during fetal life the air sacs are collapsed and full of fluid, not air. They are not used in earnest until birth has taken place.

The full structural development of the lung air sacs is complete by about twenty-four weeks of fetal life. When the formation of both the blood vessels and air sacs is completed, the lungs are structurally capable of supporting life outside the uterus. Before twenty-four weeks or so, life outside the uterus is not possible. Even at twenty-four weeks, although the major anatomical structures required for breathing air are now formed, the lining of the lung is not fully mature. In particular, it lacks the ability to form the low surface tension air-to-water interface that allows the air sacs to remain open at all times.

As with so many other organ systems, we can see the beginnings of the nervous system in the fourth week of embryonic life. The human nervous system was everyone's first computer. It is certainly the most personal of computers. It has its own unique personal

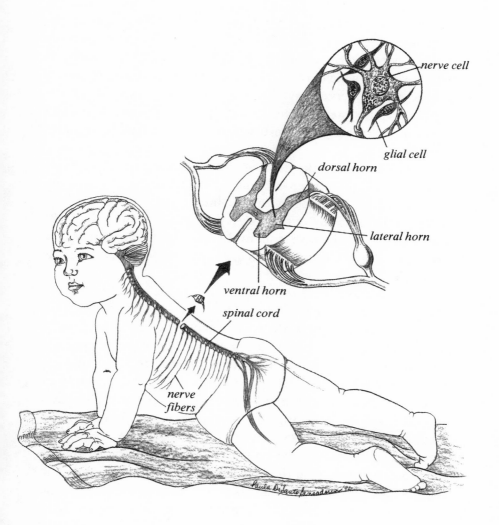

FIGURE 3.3
Diagrammatic representation of the central nervous system (the brain and spinal cord) and
the peripheral nervous system.

internal program tucked away inside the genetic material provided by the mother's ovum and the father's sperm. Neurologists and neurophysiologists divide the nervous system into the central nervous system (the brain and spinal cord), and the peripheral nervous system, which brings information through incoming nerves into the central nervous system and conducts messages from the central nervous system through outgoing nerves to the muscles and glands. These messages are instructions on what actions they must undertake.

By the fourth week the nervous system consists of a long tube, the neural tube, that runs nearly the full length of the embryo from head to tail. In keeping with the importance of its eventual function, the nervous system develops more slowly than the cardiovascular or digestive systems. In fact, development of critical structures in the brain and spinal cord continues for several months after birth.

The nervous system is composed of nerve cells and supporting cells of several types collectively called glial cells. The nerve cell is a "touchy, feely" type of cell always wanting to make contact with its brother and sister nerve cells. It has a particular ability to put out extensions in all directions. Some of these are very small and are called dendrites. In addition to possessing vast numbers of dendrites many nerve cells have one long extension called an axon. Dendrites can make contact with other nerve cells close by, but the axon allows a nerve cell to make contact with another nerve cell a long way off. The longest axons in the human body can be as long as four feet. They run from the base of the spine all the way to the brain. We are only now beginning to learn what factors control the growth of axons and how their growth is directed along the right track so that the correct connections are made.

The early organization and development of the nervous system into distinct regions can most easily be seen in the spinal cord. By the twelfth week, the primitive spinal cord has developed so that the thin innermost lining surrounds the central canal, which is filled with fluid. On the outside of the cord is the white matter, which contains the fibers of the nerve cells as they run up and down the cord. Some fibers run the full length of the cord, others connect different parts of the cord. Between the fibers are the nerve cells, or grey matter. The grey matter is divided into three discrete areas each of which often has a triangular shape, giving rise to them being named "horns." The dorsal horn is composed of cells that process incoming sensory information. The ventral horn contains cells that will send out messages to the muscles. There is also a small lateral horn, only present in those parts of the spinal cord that send out axons to glands such as digestive glands, and muscle cells in the heart, blood vessels, and digestive system that we cannot control voluntarily. This involuntary part of the nervous system is called the autonomic nervous system

The autonomic nervous system plays a key role in adults in regulating automatic, reflex responses that regulate the cardio-vascular and digestive systems. In the fetus the autonomic nervous system is critical to his ability to conduct complex cardiovascular responses to protect himself from life-threatening situations. One such dangerous situation is lack of oxygen. Later, we shall see how amazingly capable the fetus is in taking effective action to conserve available oxygen and energy sources for the brain when either or both of these sources is restricted.

Outside the spinal cord, cushioning it and the nerve rootlets as they enter and leave the spinal cord, is the very specialized cerebrospinal fluid (CSF for short). CSF is mostly produced deep within the brain in the same central canal that is in the spinal cord. This central canal runs the full length of the developing neural tube. At one point, near the junction of the brain and spinal cord, there is a hole through which the CSF escapes to the outside of the brain and spinal cord. It can then pass up and down the spine, cushioning the brain as well as the spinal cord. If there is an infection of the brain, spinal cord, or the cell layers around them, the physician can insert a small needle into the CSF space and take out a CSF fluid sample. In the laboratory this CSF sample can be tested to determine the nature of the infection or other related problem.

The brain arises from the front end of the neural tube. It will come as no surprise that the maturation of the brain is far more complex than the maturation of the spinal cord. However, the underlying principles of differentiation of the nerve cells and fibers are the same. The brain develops by a carefully programmed sequence of foldings, indentations, and outpushings that occur at breathtaking speed. Even in the very primitive embryo we can recognize three basic divisions of the developing brain, the forebrain, midbrain, and hindbrain. The central cavity filled with fluid is called the ventricular system. At its peak late in pregnancy, the developing brain is producing one hundred thousand nerve cells per minute. The brain will contain ten billion nerve cells by the time of birth. The formation of these cells requires information from the genetic code housed within the dividing cells. The brain also draws on information from the fetus' own environment and activities. After birth the very process of walking helps to develop the neuromuscular coordination necessary to enable a toddler to walk. This same process of activity-dependent development appears to happen before birth. Modern neuroscience has clearly shown the importance of interaction with the environment on brain development. Consequently in cases of premature birth the baby must develop within the alien environment of an intensive care unit (see Chapter 15). Neonatologists are much concerned with finding the best way to make up for the premature baby's early loss of his intrauterine fetal environment.

In the developing brain the middle layer of cells gives rise to the nerve cells and the outer layer to the fibers, much the same way as in the spinal cord. Different groups of nerve cells develop different functions. The dorsal (back) portion of the middle layer provides nerve cells whose functions are to gather information while the ventral (front) nerve cells are generally executive in function. However, while in the spinal cord the nerve cells remain clearly separate from the fibers, in the brain the arrangements become much more complex. Nerve cells migrate out into the white matter, moving energetically among the fibers over vast areas of the brain. This migration of nerve cells to the outside is particularly prominent in the cerebral cortex, the outer layer of the enlarged front end of the brain, which is responsible for many of the higher nervous functions such as sight, movement, and reasoning. As a result, the grey matter of the brain is on the outside over the fibers, not beneath them as in the spinal cord. In some places the nerve cells stay in the central areas in little clusters among the fibers performing specific functions. These clusters are called nuclei. This choice of the word "nucleus" to describe a group of nerve cells serving a particular function, or small group of functions, is somewhat confusing as the same word is also used for the nucleus of each individual cell. It is, however, a word that has special importance, as will be discovered when we look at the origin of the fetal signals that give rise to the birth process.

The group of nerve cells in a nucleus are best thought of as a small colony dedicated to a particular function or a group of functions. Thus we see that in the hypothalamus, a very primitive part of the brain that can be seen even in animals low down in the evolutionary scale, there are many cells that produce and secrete the hormone oxytocin. Oxytocin is secreted into the blood by pregnant women at the time of labor and delivery. It acts as a signal to the muscle cells of the uterus, causing them to contract. The supraoptic and paraventricular nuclei are the two major hypothalamic nuclei containing oxytocin. In addition to oxytocin, nerve cells in these nuclei produce many other chemicals that provoke activity in other cells. Chemicals that pass messages from one cell to another are called transmitters. Each of the functions they provoke is highly sophisticated and it is a feature of the success of the higher mammals that they have developed an extraordinary array of complex functions. Each function by itself is complex. Interacting together as they do, the end result is a truly awesome capability of mental and motor skills.

The brain owes it capabilities to a large extent to the development of many different nerve cells with specific functions. The prolific number of cells produced by division of the primitive nerve cells, however, enormously increases its capabilities. The human nervous system contains two hundred billion cells. The complexity of the nervous system becomes awe-inspiring when we consider not just the number of cells but the multitude and variety of their synaptic interconnections. It is this astronomical number and range of connections that enable the brain to perform the wide diversity of tasks of which it is capable. The myriad connections also permit extraordinary fine-tuning of function. Neuro-physiologists have shown that while the passage of an impulse down an individual axon is either "go" or "no go," each nerve cell acts like a small adding machine, summing up positive and negative inputs from other nerve cells and chemicals circulating in the blood, and deciding just how much activity it wishes to perform.

Each nerve cell has all the genetic information that every other cell in the body possesses. It used to be thought that each nerve cell produces and secretes only one transmitter. We now know that this simple clear-cut mode of action is inaccurate. Recent studies have shown that nerve cells, under certain circumstances, produce more than one transmitter. The ability of an individual nerve cell to produce and secrete more than one regulatory command molecule provides the potential to increase the complexity of function of the nervous system. We do not yet know precisely the circumstances under which nerve cells might secrete more than one transmitter at a time, or when they stop secreting one and secrete another. Undoubtedly, research will answer this question in the next few years. It is an exciting time. It is as if we suddenly discover that an oboe, which can only play one beautiful note at a time, after all, has the capacity to play chords.

To summarize, as the nervous system develops, myriad cells form in thousands of locations. Each location is a specific micro-environment. Each cell develops specific capabilities that are related to other cells nearby and depend on the input from the surrounding environment, both within the fetus itself and via signals from the mother. The sum total of the expertise of all these nerve cells is responsible for the infinite variety of potential, power, talent, and mental and physical capability that represents a particular individual. None of us end up exactly the same as another. Even identical twins have different intrauterine experiences such as differences in intrauterine position and blood supply. These differences will result in permanent variations that may be so subtle that they elude the testing methods we currently use and the demands placed on individuals by society. One very clear indication of these differences is the observation that identical twins vary in weight at birth by a few grams. We speak accurately when we refer to a person as an individual. Total individuality, indeed uniqueness, is the nature of the human race.

Our five senses are sight, hearing, smell, taste, and touch. They all begin to develop during fetal life. The organs and nerves that control our senses are indispensable to our ability to relate to the environment in which we live. Without the information we obtain from our sense organs, we would not know what is going on in the world around us, and consequently we could not enjoy our surroundings. This information from our sense organs allows us to make appropriate responses to life-threatening situations. It is now clear that the quality and quantity of the input from the sense organs to the nervous system plays an important role in the development and maturation of the system itself.

There are some general principles that appear to apply during the development of all sense organs, regardless of type. First, development begins early, around the fourth week, but completion of the structural differentiation, the hook-up to the nervous system and the full functional development, may not be completed until after birth. Second, the sensory elements that perceive the actual stimulus—that is to say light to the eye, sound waves to the ear, chemicals in the case of taste and smell, and temperature or pressure acting on the skin—are all modified nerve cells that have grown out from the nervous system. Third, around these sensory elements the fetus develops structures that protect the sensory element, such as the tough casing around the eye. It also develops mechanisms to increase the efficiency of sensation such as the trumpet-shaped ear for collecting sound, or the lens of the eye for focusing the image.

A general point about the development of sense organs during life before birth is well worth consideration. The sense organs may not have too much of a role to play while the fetus is in the uterus, but he may need them the moment he is born. Without a well-developed ability to sense temperature changes, the newborn baby will not be able to regulate his body temperature. In the uterus he does not have to undertake this task. His mother regulates her body temperature, and hence the temperature of the environment

in which the fetus lives. This is an excellent example of the fetus
having to develop the ability to deal with a challenge he has yet to
experience.

If we look at the development of the eye we see that in the fourth
week of embryonic life a pouch pushes out from the developing
forebrain on both sides. In the fifth week this pouch, the optic
vesicle, indents to form a cup. The inner surface of the cup contains
the nerve cells that will form the light-sensitive cells of the retina.
They are connected to other nerve cells in the stalk that pushed out
from the brain. This stalk will form the optic nerve, whose role it is
to relay to the brain the information generated as light lands on the
retina. A thick layer of tough connective tissue forms around the
eye giving the eyeball its characteristic shape and acting as a
protection for this vital organ. Incorporated within the eyeball is
the lens.

The differentiation and development of the outer layer of cells or
epithelium that give rise to the lens is programmed by the arrival of
the optic cup beneath it. This differentiation is an excellent
example of one tissue talking to another. The optic vesicle induces
the formation of the lens. Thus we can see that the correctly
programmed arrival of one tissue will critically affect the
differentiation of another. By the tenth week of fetal life the eye is
structurally well formed, but the nerve connections are still
developing. In other words, although a rudimentary eye is present,
the connections to the brain have not formed so the fetus does not
"see" at this stage.

Nerve fibers from the retina are the first stage on a pathway that
transfers information from the eye to a specific region of the
posterior part of the cerebral cortex known as the visual cortex. It
is in the visual cortex that we do most of our complex analysis of
visual information. From studies conducted in adult animals, we
know that the visual cortex is laid out so that it resembles a map of
the world we see. It has been found that if one eye of a newborn
animal is not functioning properly, the lack of incoming information
from that eye to the visual cortex alters the development of the
visual cortex. Thus normal function of the eye is vital to normal
development of function of the visual components of the brain.
Existing evidence suggests that this is so in the human.

In the development of the next main sensory function—hearing—the auditory nerve grows out from the hindbrain. It supplies fibers to the structures that form both the organ of hearing and the organ of balance within the ear. The ear is not fully developed until the fourth month. Even when the ear appears structurally mature, the central connections are still developing. Electrical recordings made from the brain of the fetus in response to sound suggest that maturation continues throughout fetal life.

As with so many other organs, it is the fourth week that sees the beginnings of the fetal reproductive and urinary tracts. In the adult these structures have an obvious and very close relationship. It is not surprising that their embryonic and fetal development are very closely interrelated. By the fourth week of embryonic life, a series of structures that resemble the kidneys of fish and amphibians develop on the back wall of the abdomen of the developing fetus. The first pair of kidneys disappears without trace. The second pair eventually becomes part of the male reproductive tract and disappears almost without trace in females. The third pair of developing kidneys becomes the permanent adult kidneys in both sexes. This kidney is connected on each side to the developing bladder by the ureter.

At the very earliest stages of embryonic life, the embryo has made no commitment to developing either in the female or the male fashion. The structures that will form either a testis or ovary contain a central area, called the medulla, and an outer area called the cortex. In the first week or two of embryonic life, even an experienced microscopist cannot tell whether the primitive reproductive structures (the gonad) in any particular embryo are going to become a testis or an ovary. Although we cannot see the genes, the information on which that choice will be made is contained within the genetic programming of the embryo—within the chromosomes.

Humans have twenty-three pairs of chromosomes, including one pair of sex chromosomes. In the female the sex chromosomes are similar in shape and are called the x-chromosomes. In males there is one x-chromosome and one y-chromosome. In 1990, some British researchers showed that a single gene on the male y-chromosome provides instructions that eventually result in the primitive gonad differentiating as a testis. In the testis, the central medulla develops into very thin tubes in which sperm will begin to form and the outer cortex becomes a tough protective coat.

In the absence of this male influence located on the y-chromosome, the gonad develops as an ovary. It is an underlying rule in the development of sexual differentiation that the female pattern forms when there is no male influence. There is no specific influence creating the female reproductive structures. The sexual organs are originally capable of forming either the male or female reproductive organs. If the male factor is present, the system develops in the male fashion. If the male factor is absent, the female pattern develops.

The early embryo has two separate duct systems available from which to form the reproductive tract, a male duct system and a female duct system. If a testis is developing, it secretes an inhibitory factor that causes the unwanted female duct system to disappear, or regress. This compound is a small protein. In females, because the testis is absent, the female duct does not disappear. Instead it develops to form the uterus and vagina. Again the general rule manifests itself: there is no need for a specific regulatory factor to be present for the genetic codes present in the female reproductive system to show themselves.

The patterns and rules of development of the reproductive tract were originally worked out by Professor Alfred Jost from the Collège de France in Paris. He showed that if he removed both testes from developing male rabbits, the female ducts did not regress but developed normally. If he only removed the testis from one side of the male fetus, the female duct regressed on the side where the testis remained, but developed on the side from which he had removed the testis. These elegant studies showed that duct regression factor acts locally, and not by gaining access to the fetal blood and circulating around the body. It is what is known as a paracrine regulator. Later, we will see that similar mechanisms exist to program sexual differentiation of brain development.

In summary, we have seen how the major fetal organ systems develop. We have followed some cells as they divide and migrate

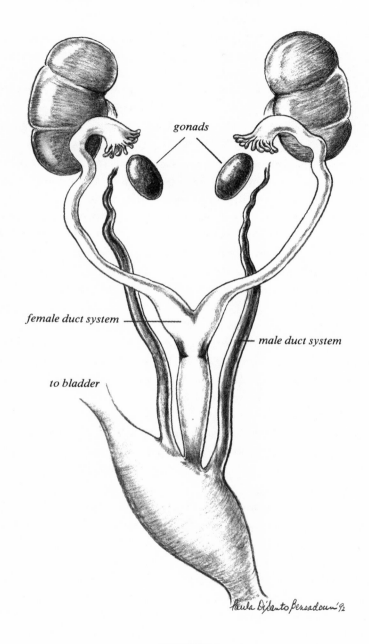

FIGURE 3.4

Sex differentiation. The early embryo has the primitive structures that can give rise to both the male and female duct systems. For clarity, the bladder has been removed.

around the developing embryo. In the midst of all the cellular activity there must be regulatory mechanisms that produce the required form and interrelationship of the many types of cells in the different organs. We have had a hint of this regulatory communication in the way the lens of the eye and the retina interrelate. There are many marvels that we have not addressed. For example, how do muscles and tendons grow together so that they are inserted into the correct little bumps on growing bones and so produce the appropriate system of levers for walking, standing, running, singing, and breathing? Opposing sets of muscles are coordinated in their development so that the correct nerves wire up to each. The muscles pull against bones that move at the joints. Muscles, bones, and joints comprise a beautifully developed set of levers. These capabilities are all products of that extraordinary burgeoning and interrelationship of cells that takes place in embryonic development under the controlling guidance of the genetic code.

During embryonic and fetal life, human development appears to recapitulate our evolutionary history. At one stage the developing embryo possesses a complete set of slits in the pharynx that look very much like the gill-slits of fish. While in human development these structures rapidly degenerate, or are converted into other structures, in fish they continue to develop and are used for extracting oxygen from the surrounding water. Until eight weeks of age the human embryo has a vestigial tail, but this is then lost. These are examples of a general law of embryonic and fetal development first put forward by Gavin De Baer in the last century. This law states that the embryonic development of the individual recapitulates the evolutionary history of the species. The yolk sac, the gill-slits, the tail, and the primitive kidney structures are all reminders of our evolutionary ancestors.

The correct completion of the overall program of development requires cells to be able to talk to each other, to give each other instructions, and to monitor how everything is progressing. Research conducted in the last twenty years has brought an explosion in our knowledge of the language cells use to regulate their interactions.

Chapter 4

CELL TALK

To do good and communicate, forget not...
The Epistle of Paul to the Hebrews, Chapter 13, v. 16

Good, the more communicated, more abundant grows.
John Milton, *Paradise Lost*

Parents provide the blueprint for construction of a new person. It is then the environment that modifies the way this blueprint unfolds. Every cell in the fetus contains within its nucleus the complete genetic code passed on by its mother and father. The genes in the cell's nucleus are the molecular basis of inheritable characteristics. They are the computer software from which the fetus will eventually unfold his own master plan for development. The software is written down within the genes in a very precise, yet simple, code. Every human has about one hundred thousand genes located on their forty-six chromosomes. The chromosomes are present at all times within the nucleus of the cell, but only become visible at the time the cell prepares to divide into two daughter cells. For every function, each cell contains a gene from each parent. Prior to division, each gene is copied so that the dividing cell contains two copies of the gene it received from the mother, and two copies of the father's gene. Then when the cell divides, one copy of the father's and one of the mother's gene are distributed to the nucleus of each of the two daughter cells.

Using powerful x-rays pictures can be produced of the structure of the gene. Francis Crick, James Watson, and their colleagues working in Cambridge, England in the 1950s demonstrated that genes are made up of a double helix of two strands of deoxyribonucleic acid (DNA). Because of the ingenious structure of DNA it is unique to each individual. The identity of the DNA is in a sense the identity of the person.

Each molecule of DNA is actually a double strand of units like two strings of pearls wound around each other to form the double helix. The strands are made up of four distinct types of molecules: adenine (A), thymine (T), guanine (G), or cytosine (C). Each strand of DNA is made up of several hundred of these blocks. While the individual components are simple, it is the order of the blocks that provides the complexity of the code.

The fundamental problem facing a cell that needs to divide is how to copy the DNA in its nucleus so that each daughter cell has all the inherited software—the same DNA structure. Until recently the ability of the cell to produce a perfect copy of the genetic DNA has been one of life's most intimate mysteries. This mystery is now rapidly being unravelled. The system that nature has evolved to replicate the DNA code is awesome in its simplicity. As the two strands that make up the DNA double helix wind around each other, the blocks are very precisely paired off opposite each other, one on each strand. A is always placed opposite T and C is always opposite G. The reason for this is that T and C are short and of the same length while A and G are long and of the same length. Thus, when T on one strand of DNA is opposite A on the other, the two strands are kept apart at the same distance as when C is opposite G. So the two strands wind around each other as a perfect double helix, with the spacing between the blocks kept absolutely constant.

The pairing has two advantages. First, it ensures that each strand of the double helix winds correctly around the other. The two strands are complementary to each other, fitting like two matched pieces of a jigsaw puzzle. It is as if the gene knows that opposite an A there must be a T and opposite a G there must be a C. Second, this precise pairing of one strand with the opposite strand provides a very simple system that enables the double helix to reproduce itself. At the time of cell division the attachment between the paired building blocks loosens and the two strands unwind and separate.

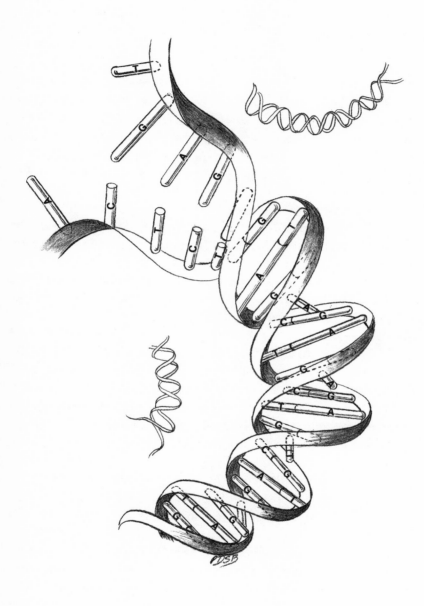

FIGURE 4.1
The DNA double helix unwinding.

The A, T, C, and G building blocks now stand out exposed without a partner. There are now two separate strands, strand I and strand II. They are exactly complementary to each other. Where there is an A on I there is a T on II. The order of the building blocks on the exposed surface is a pattern that dictates exactly how the new copies of the double helix will form. On each strand an A attaches to a new T and a C to a new G. As a result two new double helices are formed. This replicating system is exquisite in its simplicity and power. Because of the pairing of the building blocks the two strands twist around each other as the double helix forms again.

It is errors in this replicating process that on occasion give rise to mutations. These mutations in fact will provide a new instruction. The new sequence of building blocks may or may not make sense to the cell. If the mutation is large it is often lethal. It is as if a new, incomprehensible word has been introduced into the instruction language.

What the genetic DNA code does fundamentally is to provide a manufacturing template, or pattern block, on which proteins can be synthesized or reproduced. Proteins are one of the three basic types of molecule in the human body—the others are fat and carbohydrates. Molecules are the physical stuff that animals are actually made of, the units of construction. Proteins play key roles both as structural units that make up the framework of cells as well as enzymes, the key regulators of the cell's various production lines. Enzymes are very specialized proteins that increase the rate of chemical reactions in the body without being used up or altered themselves.

Each gene carries the code for one particular protein. Each protein is made up of a string of amino acids. Amino acids are the building blocks of proteins. They are relatively small molecules that contain up to three nitrogen atoms, eleven carbon atoms, and fifteen hydrogen atoms. There are twenty different amino acids in the proteins contained within our bodies. Each amino acid has a specific name. Examples are tyrosine and phenylalanine. It is amazing that a genetic code with only four different blocks can provide enough information on the sequence in which to string the twenty amino acids.

The production of proteins takes place within the outer envelope of the cell but outside the nucleus. This space is filled with a soup-like collection of molecules and structures. It is called the cytoplasm. It is as if the cell wants to protect its software program, keeping it securely locked away in the nucleus. So the nucleus sends out a precisely coded message into the cytoplasm. This message tells the production machinery in the cytoplasm to start producing more protein. To do this, DNA is copied to produce a single strand of a related molecule ribonucleic acid (RNA), which is made up of four blocks that are the same as those in DNA but with uracil (U) instead of thymine (T). A specific sequence of three of these building blocks—a triplet—in a strand represents a single amino acid. Because any one of the four building blocks can be in any of the three positions, there are four times four times four (or sixty-four) potential triplet groupings of the four blocks. Thus there are more than enough combinations of triplets to represent the twenty amino acids. In fact some amino acids are represented by more than one triplet code. For example, both UAU (uracil-adenine-uracil) and UAC (uracil-adenine-cytosine) will tell the cell's synthetic machinery to string a tyrosine amino acid. UUU tells the production line to string a phenylalanine. When the code in the nucleus is being read from the RNA to produce a protein, each sequence of three blocks in the RNA gives a specific instruction to string the appropriate amino acid on the protein string as it is forming. In this way complex proteins containing hundreds of amino acids are strung together. Because the DNA strand is several hundred triplets long, there is an almost infinite sequence of triplets. Each protein will have a unique order and shape. The whole process of protein production is a carefully designed amplification system in which a precise code is maintained. A single DNA molecule is used to make many RNA molecules each of which retains the pattern of the DNA's message. Each RNA molecule can then be used as the template to build hundreds of molecules of a unique protein made up of a string of amino acids in a specific order. In this way, one DNA molecule can be the cell's memory that allows the production of thousands of protein molecules that are needed by the cell each day as enzymes or structural components.

There are two separate, and to some extent conflicting, features in the developmental program of cells. These are growth and differentiation.

Growth of tissues takes place when individual cells in the tissue grow and then divide to produce more cells. Growth of each individual cell depends on the ability of the cell to manufacture more of all the components that make up the cell. As the components accumulate, the cell enlarges.

Eventually the cell will have to stop growing or divide into two because as the cell grows its surface area gets smaller in relation to its volume. The surface area of the cell is critical because it is through the surface that the cell gets its nutrients. When the cell grows past a certain size the relatively smaller surface area can no longer adequately cater to the cell's needs while at the same time carry away waste products.

There is a basic cell cycle that cells go through as they grow and then divide to form two cells of the same type. Growth and early divisions of cells following fertilization have been extensively studied using frogs' eggs and early embryos. The frog's egg is so loaded with energy stores that a rapid succession of divisions can occur without any production, or synthesis, of new cellular building blocks. The only new materials that need to be synthesized between the early divisions are the DNA molecules, which are the instructional blueprints for each new cell. In the developing frog embryo, cells divide every thirty minutes or so. From one initial cell, after thirty minutes there are two; after one hour, four; after two hours, sixteen. By just six hours there are four thousand ninety-six! Remember, after all that activity, the developing frog is no larger—no new tissues have been synthesized. It has just split up into many more cells, but each of them has the blueprint in its original form securely locked in its information bank ready for use when the moment arrives.

In these early divisions, the central purpose is to generate more cells in preparation for the growth of all the tissues of the body: skin, muscle, brain, etc. Each cell division has occurred so rapidly that there has been very little time to grow. Eventually cells in the tissues where growth is important begin to spend more time in the growth phase than in the division phase of the cell cycle. The relative activity of the growth and division phases of the cycle vary greatly from one situation to another depending on the nature of the cell. The duration of the cell cycle in human embryos may be as short as one hour. In adult liver cells the cycle lasts a year. Some cells, such as nerve cells, eventually lose the ability to divide.

In the laboratory, when extracts of cells in the process of dividing are injected into cells that are in the resting phase between divisions, the recipient cells are stimulated to divide. This seems to suggest that messenger molecules within the cell are controlling the drive to divide. The production of these regulators of cell division is controlled by the blueprint within the nucleus of the cell. We still do not know what switches on production of the regulatory messengers that stimulate division.

Equally mysterious is how cells become differentiated in function when they all arise from the single fertilized egg. Even though the initial daughter cells of the egg look very much alike, very early on we can detect differences in capabilities. After three divisions there are eight cells in a mammalian embryo. If we separate one of these eight cells and grow it alone it will develop differently from the other seven. In the process of differentiation, a cell focuses on developing some of its capabilities to the exclusion of others. One cell commits itself to becoming a nerve cell, another a muscle cell, for the rest of its life. The basic cell types are called stem cells. It is by the differentiation of the stem cells that new or replacement tissues with specific functions are formed. Once the decision is made and the differentiation complete there is usually no going back.

We do not yet know how the blueprint lodged in the initial single fertilized egg actually handles all its different tasks. However, many techniques to help answer this question have been developed and research groups around the world are hard at work. One area of study involves the mapping of all the divisions of a small worm that is composed of only nine hundred fifty-nine cells. Even the study of an organism with this limited number of cells is a very complex task. The worm under study needs to produce the same complex range of different tissues as mammalian organisms. It has the full range of cell types: muscle cells, brain cells, and skin cells. It is the relatively small number of cells that makes the worm much easier to study. Of course, eventually we will need to see how the principles discovered in these non-mammalian control systems apply to mammals, including ourselves; that is a whole new area of study in itself.

It appears that the differentiation of cells involves information and commands received from neighboring cells in addition to the use of instructions in the blueprint. This instructional input to a cell from its neighbors is not so surprising. The neighboring cells all got to where they are because of their own blueprint, and they each have something to say to the cells next to them about the final outcome. The final body shape of the adult and its proper function will depend on all cells having made the right decisions. The science of cell biology looks at the social constraints imposed by cells on themselves and each other. Nothing exists in a vacuum. By its very existence each cell has an effect on its neighbors. The body is like a society composed of a large number of varied cells eventually allocated to different tissues to perform specialized jobs. Successful development of the embryo depends on how well these cells communicate with each other during development.

Cells have their own unique way of communicating with one another. Humans communicate with each other by several methods that affect the sense organs of the other individual. We talk and are heard; we make gestures and use body language that is seen; we touch and are felt; we also pass signals to others by our body odors. When cells wish to communicate with each other they use two major mechanisms, nerve impulses and messenger chemicals. This information from other cells is obtained from molecules that attach to specific receptors on the outer surface of the cell and alter its activity.

Nerve impulses are carried in nerve fibers. One major function of nerve fibers is to instruct muscle cells to contract and do the job they were designed to do. Electrical impulses pass all the way along the nerve fiber to the end. There, the nerve fiber secretes a specific transmitter. The transmitter diffuses across a very narrow junction, called a synapse. The synapse separates the nerve fiber from the muscle cell. Like all molecules, the transmitter molecule has a special shape. This unique shape allows the transmitter, and only the transmitter, to fit like a key into a lock on the muscle cell membrane. The lock into which it fits is called a receptor. When the correct fit is made between the lock and key, their interaction sets up a chain of reactions within the muscle cell. As a result, the muscle fiber contracts.

Nerve fibers are an excellent long-distance signalling mechanism, but they have limitations, too. They are like the telephone network before the days of satellite communications. Nerve fibers cannot send messages to cells with which they are not directly connected. On the other hand, the big advantage of the nervous system is that it transmits instructions very quickly. Some nerves transmit messages at the rate of up to one hundred meters per second. When the body wants to respond to urgent situations the advantages of speed overcome the limitations of restricted distribution.

The second mechanism for cell communication does not require nerve fibers. Some cells in organs known collectively as endocrine organs, or glands, produce specific instructional molecules called hormones (from the Greek word hormao: to excite). The function of the endocrine glands is to manufacture and secrete their hormone product at specific times and under specific situations. Hormone molecules are secreted by the endocrine cells directly into the bloodstream to circulate around the body. Endocrine glands are always especially well supplied with blood vessels so that they can easily discharge their messages into the blood. The endocrine method of signalling is slow compared with the nervous system. Its advantage is that the hormone message can get to anywhere the blood goes.

Hormone messenger molecules circulate around the body in the blood. When they reach the tissue whose activity they are designed to modify, the hormone molecule attaches to the cell surface of its target. Only the cells specifically targeted possess the right receptors to bind the hormone. In this way the hormone can chose the exact cell it talks to. Just as with the transmitter at the synaptic junction between nerves and muscle cells, the interaction between the hormone and the receptor initiates a complex set of reactions within the target cell. Hormone molecules can give orders to either increase a particular cellular function or decrease it. An example of this is progesterone, which is a hormone produced by the placenta. It has a general inhibitory effect on the ability of the uterine muscle cells to contract; in contrast, estrogens, also produced by the placenta, have the effect of stimulating the uterine muscle to contract. Both these hormones have important roles to play in the process of birth as we shall see in Chapters 12 and 13.

In addition to sending long-distance messages carried by nerve fibers or hormones, cells indulge in local small talk. Studies over the last twenty years have identified regulatory signalling messenger molecules that do not need to get into the blood stream to modify processes in adjacent cells. These molecules are secreted by cells into their immediate neighborhood. They bind to receptors on nearby cells and alter the function of these neighbors. These local regulatory molecules are said to act in a paracrine fashion, whereas endocrine hormone messengers are secreted into the blood. Paracrine regulation is a local conversation, one cell talking to neighboring cells and giving them information and instructions. The endocrine hormone messengers, in contrast, carry on long-distance conversations. The chemical structure of paracrine regulators is as varied as the structure of hormones. Both groups act on the surface receptors to influence fundamental activities of their target cells. On the surface of most cells there are receptors to many hormones as well as to paracrine regulatory molecules from adjacent cells present in the fluid surrounding the cell. The final level of activity of each cell will depend on the balance of all the stimulatory and inhibitory regulators acting on it.

There is one major feature of the development of conversation between cells that has a real human parallel: it's no use talking if no one is listening, and it is no use talking in a language that the listener does not understand. Successful conversation between cells requires the recipient cell to have the correct receptors. Thus, factors that regulate the type and number of receptors on the cell membrane will influence the conversation. As we shall see in Chapter 12, some hormones alter the number of receptors that a target cell might have for receiving other, different hormones. At one time in its life a cell may have only a few receptors available for adrenaline, for example. Then, at a later stage in development, steroid hormones may stimulate the production of adrenaline receptors on the cell surface so that the cell can then respond to messages delivered as packets of adrenaline. It is as if the steroid hormone has taught the cell in question a new language or to use another image, as though it has laid in another radiophone for incoming calls.

How a transmitter, hormone, or other regulatory molecule binds to the cell membrane causing an altered function of that cell is another intriguing question. There are several mechanisms, but they are very similar in all cell types. In many instances there is a change in the electrical potential that exists across the surface of the cell. In nerves and muscles the change will cause the passage of an electrical impulse across the surface of the cell. In nerves this impulse will pass down to the junction with the next cell, cause release of a transmitter, and alter the activity of the next cell. The conversation has continued; two cells have interacted on behalf of the whole body. If it is a muscle cell whose membrane potential has been changed, the muscle will contract.

In other cells, activation of the receptor leads to a cascade of consequences. In some cells, genes are switched on thereby altering the function of the DNA. As a result, the cell changes what it is doing. In other cases the effect is to activate within the cell specific regulatory proteins called enzymes, thereby stimulating the manufacturing processes going on in the cell.

The mechanisms cells use to interact are very old in evolutionary terms. A common one used in regulating cell function is a small molecule called cyclic adenosine monophosphate—cyclic AMP for short. In several different types of cells the interaction of the message with the cell surface receptor results in the production of the regulatory molecule cyclic AMP within the cell. Cyclic AMP has been around for a very long time, and is used by cells in a very primitive slime mold to signal to each other. These slime molds live on the ground in dark, impenetrable forests. Usually they exist as individual cells feeding on nutrients in the ground moisture and dividing every few hours. If local food supplies get short, the separate cells begin to secrete cyclic AMP. This is the signal to stop dividing and get together to form a worm-like structure that can crawl around looking for better supplies of food. The worm leaves a slimy trail and thus gets its name, slime mold. Cyclic AMP is a very old "word" in the language cells use as an instruction to change their activities.

The human embryo, in its very early development, does not have a nervous system or a blood system to carry hormones around from endocrine cells to target tissues, so all cell-to-cell interactions are paracrine. Nevertheless, the mechanism of conversation between cells is still the same and many of the same regulator molecules are used. At all stages of growth and differentiation, cells need information and instruction in order to make the correct responses to their environment. Each cell needs to know where it is and what its function should be. In the early embryo the only information the cell needs is of a very general nature like: "Which end is the head and which is the tail?" Later the cells need to know their location more precisely. Are they in the heart, or the liver, for example? Parallels can be drawn yet again with human society. Early in the life of the embryo, all cells must be able to range far and wide and carry out every conceivable function, just like the resourceful pioneers in a new land. Later, as their society becomes more sophisticated, skills are specialized. Each individual cell hones some skills, loses some, and usually chooses one specific place to settle down.

The computer program that directs the development process must keep the factors responsible for cell division (growth) and cell specialization (differentiation) working along the appropriate time path, giving the correct emphasis to each of these two conflicting but complementary activities. It has to work with amazing accuracy. Using the program appropriately, the body needs to generate all the necessary cell types in their correct numbers and in the appropriate places. Each cell influences the development of nearby cells. This fact can be demonstrated in the laboratory at critical periods of development by killing individual cells using a focused laser light beam narrow enough to kill a single cell only two thousandths of a millimeter in diameter. When this is done the development of nearby cells is often critically altered.

One important group of paracrine regulators are the growth factors. The pituitary gland is an endocrine gland located underneath the brain just behind the eyes. For many years it has been known that the pituitary gland secretes a protein hormone, growth hormone, into the blood. Individuals who secrete too much growth hormone in early life can end up as giants. If the excessive growth hormone secretion is the result of a tumor that develops late in life after the long bones have stopped growing, a different picture is seen; only the hands, feet, and jaw bone are able to respond by growing excessively. The clinical condition is then known as acromegaly. The patient is normal in height but the lower jaw protrudes and the hands and feet are grossly enlarged.

Growth hormone produces its effects via intermediaries, not directly. When young mice are injected with growth hormone, the parts of their limbs that are still cartilage grow rapidly, producing gigantism. However, if the cartilage cells are taken out of the body and grown in a dish with added growth hormone, the cartilage cells do not grow faster. It is now clear that growth hormone acts on almost every type of cell in the body stimulating them to produce specific growth factors that then cause other cells in the body to grow. Thus, if blood from a mouse that was injected with growth hormone is placed in the dish with the cartilage cells, the growth rate of the cartilage cells increases. This is because growth hormone worked on various cells in the body causing them to produce the growth factors. The growth factors were released into the blood and so blood from these animals treated with growth hormone can cause growth of cartilage cells in the dish.

In other words, growth hormone works to produce growth through the intermediary action of growth factors and these act in both an endocrine and paracrine fashion. Growth factors hurry the cells that respond to them through the growth and division phases of the cell cycle. Recent studies suggest that pygmies are small because many of their cells do not respond to growth hormone by producing the right amount of a particular important growth factor.

Over twenty different growth factors have already been identified. One called nerve growth factor was discovered by pure chance. It was observed that when a particular tumor was transplanted experimentally, the tumor was suddenly invaded by nerve cells. Extracts of the tumor were shown to cause processes to grow out from nerve cells when cultured. Nerve growth factor stimulates the growth of nerve processes of some, but not all, types of nerve fibers. The nerve cells that respond to nerve growth factor are those that conduct sensory information into the central nervous system.

Another interesting and important growth factor is the one that is derived from the platelets in the blood. Platelets are small cells circulating in the blood that help to form a blood clot when the skin is damaged. This growth factor descriptively, but somewhat unimaginatively, called platelet derived growth factor (PDGF), is released when tissues bleed and blood clots. PDGF stimulates connective tissue cells to grow, divide, and repair the damaged sites. The wound-healing capabilities of the fetus and newborn are very much greater than those of adults and the elderly. If we could find out why fetal cells are so good at wound-healing much might be done to improve tissue repair after trauma or burns for people of all ages. The discovery of growth factors in the last decade has opened up new ideas about how cells interact. From the practical point of view, improving our knowledge about growth factors will present marvelous opportunities for the treatment of spinal injuries, various types of dwarfism, and many other damaging conditions.

The nervous system is the only major system in the body that lacks the ability to repair and replace itself following injury. We need to know more about how growth factors function so that we can apply this knowledge to spinal injuries, brain-scarring after neurosurgery, and congenital defects.

Cells in the body are surrounded by a scaffolding, or matrix, of molecules that they and their neighboring cells secrete. This matrix is not permanent nor are cells randomly placed on it. The matrix is a constantly changing, functionally important part of the tissues with an important role to play. The scaffolding is particularly important during embryonic and fetal development. The matrix contains chemicals that alter cell development, stimulate or inhibit cell migration from one place to another, determine cell shape, and hence the shape of organs, and slow down or speed up the rate of activity of the cells contained within it. The amount of matrix in different tissues varies enormously. It forms a large portion of the bulk of bone; in the brain, although the amount of matrix between the nerve cells is only a small component, it has an extremely important function. In the brain and nervous tissues the matrix forms clearly defined pathways along which the nerve processes migrate. Hence, the matrix helps to direct nerve fibers to their correct destination.

Cells are stuck together by specialized molecules called adhesion molecules, which help to determine the formation of tissues. Thus, the precise time during development that genes regulating the production of adhesion molecules are first switched on will determine whether cells continue migrating or stay put where they are. Once cells have settled down, they form junctions of various types among themselves. These junctions help to cement functional as well as structural relationships between cells. In the matrix there are long twisted connecting molecules that curl around each other to form cable-like structures. These connective tissue structures play an important role in determining the shape of tissues and organs.

Cells, like individuals and societies, have evolved many ways of talking to each other. Our ancestors left us complex instructions in our DNA code. Early cells in the embryo secrete paracrine regulators that provide information and instructions for nearby cells. Later, when the blood system has formed, hormone messengers can circulate around the body carrying instructions. Nerve fibers develop to provide point-to-point communication.

Communication between individuals has always been important for the success of our human society. It is equally so for the correct development of form and function in the developing embryo and fetus. Apart from the intellectual excitement of burgeoning knowledge regarding embryonic and fetal development, there will eventually be a great pay-off to society from a better understanding of the regulation of cell growth and differentiation. The aging process ultimately affects us all. Cancer is an all-too-common tragedy that afflicts many people. Both aging and cancer are the result of normal and abnormal function within the cell. The instructional program within the cell may go wrong either because of intrinsic defects or because of pollutants from the environment. It is certain that as we learn more about the cell's regulatory program, medical science will develop useful management techniques to deal with cancerous cells. Of course, this knowledge will not come as fast as we would like. It is encouraging to remember that childhood leukemia was virtually universally fatal thirty years ago. Today many forms of leukemia can be cured. Learning more about the biology of the cell offers new hope for present and future generations.

Chapter 5

THE PLACENTA

The placenta is a go-between—between the mother and the fetus—
a separate unit made up of cells partly from the mother and partly
from the fetus. It is a self-contained package that is expelled with
the baby from the uterus at birth and is thrown away having done
its job. It is the body's only throw-away organ.

The placenta is unique. In two particular ways it is quite
different from all other organs in mammals. The only organ
formed from two individuals, the placenta possesses a fetal
component and a maternal component. This single organ formed
from two unique individuals each with a different genetic make-up
is unparalleled elsewhere in natural biology. In the laboratory it is
possible to produce animals called chimeras in which cells from
two different embryos early in development have been mixed and
allowed to grow to form an independent adult animal. However, in
the natural situation, only in the placenta do two distinct
organisms participate in the production of a single organ.

The placenta seems to break all the rules of individual identity.
Every individual has a concept of self laid down in their cells.
When foreign cells come into close contact with the individual, the

foreign cells generally constitute a challenge to the host's continued independent function. A good example is the invasion of the body by bacteria during an infection. The bacteria compete for the food resources circulating in the blood. If the body does not respond to this intrusion the bacteria will multiply and further deprive the host. During evolution all animals have developed defense mechanisms to reject and kill off foreign cells whenever they meet them within their own bodies. Collectively, these defense mechanisms constitute the immune system. The placenta, however, defying the immune system, allows two separate organisms—the fetus and the mother—to come into a close relationship.

This immune tolerance of the mother for the fetus is one of the many extraordinary features of pregnancy, and it is essential for the survival and growth of the placenta. It is now thought that many early miscarriages (pregnancy losses) are caused by the failure of the mother's immune system to tolerate the fetal tissue in the placenta. In these early miscarriages, the mother's body loses its normal tolerance of the embryo. If this happens the mother mobilizes her normal defense mechanisms used against foreign invaders. As a result the mother treats her embryo-child as a "foreign body," rejecting him. This explanation for some miscarriages is further supported by the fact that some women have repeated early pregnancy losses when the embryos that attempt to implant in their uterus are fathered by one particular partner. However, sometimes when that same woman carries embryos fathered by a different partner, the fetuses survive to normal birth. Each partner has a specific genetic make-up and it may be that a particular woman can develop an immune tolerance to fetuses from one father but not another. This fascinating area of study could be the subject of a book in its own right. The placenta has a unique ability to override the immune system, and much research is being conducted in this area in an attempt to understand why tissues reject each other. Knowledge of these processes is essential to improving the success of organ transplantation between individuals.

The other way in which the placenta is different from most other organs in mammals is that it is a completely disposable unit. The placenta has a specific set of functions to perform over a quite limited, though critical, period in the life-span of two people. It is then discarded with no adverse effects. If the placenta can be discarded, then the functions it performs must only be necessary for a specific period of time—the phase of growth and development of the fetus in the uterus. During this critical development period the functions of the placenta are vital. If birth occurs at the correct time, the newborn baby no longer needs his placenta.

When, as in the case of premature birth, the placenta is discarded too soon, the baby depends on the resources of the neonatal intensive care unit (NICU). The dedicated doctors and nurses who work in the NICU have to use modern technological systems developed by researchers to carry out the functions of the uterus and placenta. Unfortunately, we do not yet know enough about the placenta to enable us to replace its function completely for the premature baby. The NICU is not an exact substitute for the uterine environment, in large measure due to the loss of placental function. The goal of neonatologists working in the NICU is to find ways to simulate the conditions that the premature babies would have been experiencing had they remained in their mother's uterus. The effect of early placental loss is poorly understood and information is critically needed.

The primary function of the placenta is to act as the fetal lungs. The lungs are the organs through which the body absorbs and exchanges gases. In the lungs, oxygen is taken up and carbon dioxide is removed from the body. Because he is not in contact with the air in the outside world, the fetus must get his oxygen from, and pass his waste products into, his mother's blood. The placenta acts as the site of exchange. While the embryo is small no special equipment is necessary. Gas exchange can take place by simple diffusion as gases will diffuse rapidly through cell layers that are only a few cells thick. Primitive organisms composed of only a few hundred cells do not need lungs and neither does the embryo, until he exceeds the number of cells that can be supplied simply by diffusion. When the embryo grows and exceeds this size, he will need a transport system to carry oxygen and other vital compounds from the placenta to all the tissues of his body that cannot be reached by diffusion. The same transport system, the circulation of the blood, can be used to carry all the waste products away from their site of production to the placenta where they can be removed from the fetus and passed into his mother's circulation.

Another function of the placenta is to act as the kidney for the fetus. Mammalian organisms require precise control of the chemical make-up of their internal environment to carry out their sophisticated functions. Consider, for instance, the sequence of bodily functions that must be properly activated for an eagle to perceive and capture a fish swimming in a lake. From hundreds of feet up in the sky the eagle must first register the information that there is a fish moving in the lake. This information is gathered through the eagle's spectacularly acute visual system. The eagle must then pass the information along nerves to its brain, assess factors such as wind speed and speed of movement of the fish. He must then conduct his swoop along the required flight path. The complex set of functions requires electrical and other signals to function in a very precise way—just like a fighter aircraft. Just as the circuits of the fighter aircraft must all be perfectly operational, so must the circuitry of the eagle. To ensure that all the eagle's complex circuitry is functioning properly, the chemical composition of his body fluids must be very precisely regulated, to allow the electrical impulses to pass rapidly and in a coordinated sequence from the control areas of his brain to the required muscles and glands. What is a simple everyday event to the eagle is in fact a physiological miracle of complex design.

Likewise our internal environment is very precisely controlled with regard to concentration of different ions that permit electrical signals to pass around the body. However, the food we eat does not contain these ions and other compounds in exactly the composition that our body needs them. Our kidneys act to adjust the composition and concentration of these ions and other molecules by excreting some of the ions and retaining others in amounts appropriate to maintain the constancy of the internal environment. In the adult the kidneys also remove many toxic products from the blood and excrete them in the urine. These compounds secreted in the urine would be harmful if they were allowed to build up in the body. The kidney also regulates loss of water from the body in the urine. Water loss is regulated to keep the concentrations of ions in the body fluids within a very narrow range. When the cells that make up our body are short of water the kidney retains water and we pass only small amounts of very concentrated urine. If we drink a lot of water, the urine we form is very diluted. The placenta must perform these functions for the fetus.

The kidney is a principal regulator of the internal environment of the body. It either retains or excretes a wide variety of minerals according to the need to maintain the correct chemical composition of these compounds in the body. A good example is the sodium ion, whose concentration in the blood and tissue fluids is critical to a wide variety of electrical charges in the body in nerves, muscles (including the heart), and many other highly sophisticated cell functions. The amount of sodium retained by the adult kidney is regulated by a hormone named aldosterone. As seen in Chapter 4, in order for hormones to act, a complex system of cell surface receptors and intracellular messengers are required. As the fetus develops, these cellular processes gradually mature. Even at birth, especially if birth occurs prematurely, many functions of the kidney are still not fully developed. For instance, a premature baby's kidney is unable to excrete a water load if he is given too much fluid. The diet of even a baby born at the normal time must be carefully controlled to avoid exceeding the capacity of the relatively immature kidney to maintain a "constant internal environment." Mother's breast milk is the most suitable diet, most appropriate to the baby's need.

We do not know precisely how the placenta contributes to the control of the composition of the fetal body fluids. The major protection that the mother provides is to maintain her body composition within normal limits. These limits are similar to those of the fetus, thereby lessening the regulatory work that needs to be done by the placenta. However, studies have shown that when maternal body composition changes for some reason, for instance after ingestion of large volumes of water or saline, compensatory mechanisms are brought into play in the fetus. At times like this the placenta fulfills its important function of protecting the baby's environment.

It is only through the placenta that the fetus gets his nutrients—his food—so the placenta has to serve as a fetal digestive system. Providing she is eating a healthy diet, the mother's blood will contain all of the basic components that the fetus needs to build tissues and to provide energy. However, because maternal and fetal blood never come into direct contact, all of these compounds must pass through the cells that compose the placenta in order to reach the fetal blood. The placenta, therefore, performs the function of a fetal digestive system, at least the absorptive function. It is the only route by which the developing and growing fetus can get the basic constituents he needs to build his tissues. At the same time as helping the fetus by transporting nutrients such as glucose (an important sugar), the placenta also performs the function of a barrier preventing the passage of many toxins and infectious agents. Unfortunately, as the thalidomide tragedy showed, this barrier function is not one hundred percent perfect. As we will see in Chapter 10, thalidomide, a drug taken extensively by women in the 1960s to ward off the nausea of early pregnancy, crossed the placenta and produced fetal malformations. Transplacental passage of drugs-of-abuse is very harmful to the fetus as discussed later.

In the last twenty years several groups of researchers have carried out very elegant studies that have enabled precise quantification of the dietary intake of the fetal sheep in the last third of pregnancy. It is exciting to be able to add up the calories that the normally growing fetus uses at different stages of his life in the uterus. We can determine very precisely how much of the food he takes in across the placenta is used for building his tissues and how much is expended to generate energy needed to practice his breathing and limb muscle movements.

To obtain this information on the fetal energy balance, we must be able to measure the amounts of specific compounds that go across the placenta to the fetus, and simultaneously how much, if any, comes back from the fetus to the mother. Glucose is the major source of energy in the fetus as well as the adult mammal. We know that glucose molecules are going in both directions across the placenta, but there are many more molecules going from the mother to the fetus than from the fetus to the mother. We need to know the flux in each direction so that we can measure the net overall flux. By taking blood samples from four sites (the blood going into and out of the placenta on both sides) and measuring the blood flow on both sides of the placenta, these fluxes have been determined for glucose in sheep. Similar calculations can be made for utilization of other important molecules like oxygen, for example. We can determine how much is used by the uterus and how much by the fetus.

An ultrasonic detector can be placed experimentally around the common umbilical artery of a fetal sheep allowing us to measure continuously the flow of arterial blood from the fetus to the placenta. The probe works on the Doppler principle. One crystal in the flow probe sends out a wave of ultrasound of a known frequency. The sound wave is slowed down when it hits the red blood cells as they flow through the vessel. The change in speed of the ultrasound wave brings about a change in the frequency of the sound wave. It is the same principal that makes a train whistle seem to change note. The approaching whistle appears to have a higher note as it approaches and a lower note as it moves away from the listener. The pitch of the note depends upon the speed of the train. The amount of change in the frequency of the sound wave is related to the speed of the flowing blood. A second crystal receives the sound wave and a computer is used to calculate the change in the frequency of the sound produced by the flowing blood.

When you and I eat a meal, we take a large variety of food molecules into our digestive system. The digestive system, sometimes called the gut, is a tube of varying size composed of several highly specialized sections. From the mouth, the food passes down the esophagus into the stomach, where much preliminary breakdown of the food occurs. From the stomach food passes into the intestines. The first part of the intestine is called the small intestine because the diameter of the tube is smaller here than farther down the digestive system where the intestine expands and is, therefore, called the large intestine. The large intestine passes to the anus where the remnants of undigested food, cell debris that has worn away from the lining of the digestive system, and some of the secretions that were passed out into the digestive system are expelled as feces.

The small intestine is functionally very active, completing the
digestive processes begun in the stomach. The food we eat, be it
animal or plant material, is made up mostly of proteins,
carbohydrates, and fats that differ in their structure from animal to
animal or plant to plant. During the process of digestion the three
major groups of food are broken down into their basic components.
These components are glucose from carbohydrates, amino acids
from proteins, and fatty acids from fats, which are the fundamental
building blocks that will be used by the body to build its cells or are
burned to produce energy. They are then absorbed into the blood
stream so that we can make use of them to form our own
specialized molecules or burn them to give us energy. These two
processes, digestion and absorption, are carried out mostly in the
small intestine, although some absorption takes place in the large
intestine.

The basic elements of fetal nutrition are glucose, amino acids,
fats, water, mineral ions, and vitamins. Each of these compounds
passes through the placenta by a slightly different mechanism. The
placenta is made up of several layers of cells placed between the
maternal and fetal blood. Molecules that pass from mother to fetus
or fetus to mother must pass through this barrier. Transport may
be either by active processes in which the placental cells use energy
to pump the molecule across or by passive diffusion processes.
Passive diffusion does not require expenditure of energy and may
be sufficient to supply the fetus with his needs providing two
conditions are met. First, the concentration of the substance
attempting to cross the placenta must be higher in the maternal
blood than in the fetal blood so that the molecules of the substance
can diffuse down the concentration gradient, downhill as it were.
Second, no cell or tissue barrier must exist to impede the free
movement of the molecules of the substance across the placenta. If
these two conditions are met, molecules in solution will move
passively from areas of high concentration to areas of low
concentration without expenditure of energy. Drop a small amount
of black ink into a cup of water and the colored ink will diffuse
outward from the initial highly concentrated drop until the
concentration is the same throughout the cup. This is the same

process as diffusion down a concentration gradient across the placenta. Oxygen is an important example of a molecule that will pass passively across the placenta down its concentration gradient.

Glucose is present in maternal blood at a higher concentration than in fetal blood and can diffuse across the placenta into the fetal blood. The concentration gradient is continuously maintained because the fetus removes the glucose that has diffused into his blood. He either burns it to produce energy or stores it. We now know, however, that glucose crosses the placenta from mother to fetus more easily than can be accounted for by simple diffusion. The cells of the placenta contain a specialized carrier molecule called the glucose transporter that facilitates the transport of glucose from mother to fetus. Glucose transport across the placenta is therefore said to occur by facilitated diffusion. The glucose transporter acts like a little shuttle bus. Because there is a higher concentration of glucose molecules in the maternal blood than the fetal blood, the shuttle bus has more passenger molecules wanting to go from mother to fetus than in the reverse direction. Thus the overall transport of glucose across the placenta is from the maternal to the fetal side.

The placenta is a living organ and hence burns glucose to provide energy as it conducts its daily activities. Studies in experimental animals have quantified the glucose requirements of the placenta. In sheep the uterus and placenta consume up to two thirds of the glucose taken up from maternal blood in the uterine artery, leaving only one third to pass across the placenta to the fetus. This finding may not seem surprising, because the placenta is a very active tissue and will need some source of energy, but it does have some very important implications when the glucose supply to the uterus is decreased for any reason. At times of glucose shortage, the placenta can use glucose while in the process of passing it across to the fetus. As a result the fetus may be deprived of adequate amounts of glucose for his energy requirements. So when there is not enough glucose coming from the mother, the fetus may have no alternative but to start depleting his own meager energy reserves (see Chapter 10). In order to live, the placenta has to be fed just like the fetus.

Minerals such as calcium, sodium, and potassium exist in fluids in a form called ions, which carry an electric charge, either positive or negative. Several charged mineral ions are actively transported across the placenta. A good example is the iodide ion that is used by the thyroid gland. The thyroid gland needs iodide to produce the important hormone thyroxine. Iodide ions are present in the maternal blood at lower concentrations than in fetal blood. Iodide ions are pumped from the mother "uphill" across the placenta against a concentration gradient. This ability of the placenta to pump iodide uphill into the fetus protects the developing fetus should there be a shortage of iodide in his mother's diet and drinking water. Iodide shortages are common in some mountainous parts of the world. Untreated, iodide deficiency leads to hypothyroidism in adults (a disease in which there is a low level of activity of the thyroid gland), when all the body's processes are slowed down. In the adult, the consequences of hypothyroidism can usually be reversed even if they are diagnosed in a fairly advanced state. The treatment is to provide thyroid hormone to reverse the body's deficiency. If necessary, iodide can also be given to make up for the dietary deficiency. On the other hand, if the fetus is iodide-deficient at critical periods of development, irreversible damage may occur to the fetal brain and also to bone development. It is therefore extremely important that the fetus have the ability to pump as much iodide as he needs from the maternal circulation even if the mother is short of iodide in her blood.

The oxygen that the fetus obtains has diffused passively from the high concentration dissolved in the maternal blood, across the placenta, into the fetal blood. Oxygen is transported around the mother's circulation bound or attached to hemoglobin. Hemoglobin is a tough little molecule that carries oxygen: one molecule can pick up and transport four molecules of oxygen. The amount of oxygen carried by hemoglobin in the maternal blood at any one time depends on several factors:

- the oxygen content of the air the mother breathes,
- total amount of hemoglobin in the maternal blood,
- amount of carbon dioxide in maternal blood, and
- acidity of maternal blood.

The mother obtains oxygen from the atmosphere as her blood circulates through her lungs. The tissue in the maternal lungs needs to be healthy. If any disease process has decreased the surface area of normal maternal lung available for gas exchange, then oxygen uptake will be impaired. The total pressure of the air around us fluctuates only a little from day to day. The air contains several gases: oxygen comprises about one fifth, and nitrogen most of the rest. Each gas contributes what is called its partial pressure to the overall pressure of the air around. When there are other gases in the air we breathe, they reduce the proportion, or partial pressure, contributed by oxygen. The partial pressure of oxygen in the blood in the mother's arteries is directly related to the partial pressure in the air the mother breathes. When the partial pressure of oxygen in maternal blood is reduced for any reason, the amount of oxygen transported in maternal blood will decrease. Cigarette smoke contains much carbon monoxide and carbon dioxide. In very smoky atmospheres, the partial pressure of oxygen in the air may be significantly lowered. In many developing countries pregnant women spend much of their time inside poorly ventilated, confined living quarters. These confined areas are often filled with smoke from open fires that are generating lots of carbon monoxide and carbon dioxide. As a result the mother has a lowered hemoglobin saturation in her blood. Carbon monoxide binds irreversibly to hemoglobin thereby lowering the absolute amount of maternal hemoglobin available to carry oxygen. This unhealthy situation often leads to too little oxygen being delivered to the placenta, and hence to the fetus. Decreased oxygen transport across the placenta will lead to growth retardation. If the mother is also a cigarette smoker the situation is made worse. Even appreciable passive smoking from the fumes of other people's cigarettes in the air will contribute to a lowered oxygen-carrying capacity of the maternal blood.

Hemoglobin is a protein in red blood cells that picks up oxygen and carries it around the body. Hemoglobin contains iron. If the red cells in the mother's blood are short of hemoglobin (a condition called anemia), her ability to transport oxygen to all of her tissues will be impaired. Oxygen transport to the placenta also decreases.

The need for adequate concentrations of hemoglobin in maternal blood is very obvious. Unfortunately, often maternal health, and thus fetal health, is compromised because of poor maternal nutrition that has left the mother iron-deficient and hence anemic. The simplest way of improving the health of the fetus of an undernourished woman who is anemic is to provide her with the correct nutrients to return her circulating hemoglobin concentration to normal. The effect of this simple therapy in malnourished pregnant women is dramatic. It is an excellent example of how much can be done for the mother and her baby by improving general prenatal care, especially in the less advantaged sections of the community.

Just as oxygen is needed to support the burning of wood or coal in a fire, oxygen supports the chemical reactions the body uses to obtain energy. The main product of these reactions is carbon dioxide. Carbon dioxide is a very acidic compound, and is produced by all active tissues as they perform their functions. Hence, as blood passes through active tissues, the acidity of the blood rises. As a result of the work of the Danish Nobel Prize winner Niels Bohr, we know that hemoglobin will let go more oxygen into the blood as it becomes more acidic, and as a result of his work this process is called the Bohr shift. In this way more oxygen will be available to diffuse into these active tissues. The more active the tissue, the greater the amount of oxygen that will be freed up from the hemoglobin. This is a very neat system whereby hemoglobin provides more oxygen to active tissues than to inactive tissues. When oxygen leaves the hemoglobin carrier molecule, the hemoglobin becomes available to bind with carbon dioxide. In adults this carbon dioxide is carried back in the circulation to the lungs. Because carbon dioxide is present in greater concentration in the maternal pulmonary arterial blood going to her lungs than it is in the atmospheric air in the air sacs, carbon dioxide can pass down this concentration gradient and out of the maternal body. In the fetus, carbon dioxide leaves the fetal blood by crossing the placenta into the maternal circulation.

If there is not enough oxygen to support the energy-providing reactions in the cells of the fetus, they are not carried through to completion, and acidic products such as lactic acid are produced. The acidity produced by these compounds cannot be discharged by the lungs. These acids are not easily released as gases in the same way as is carbon dioxide, and must be got rid of very much more slowly across the placenta into the mother's blood stream. In a fetus that is short of oxygen these acid molecules may form faster than the placenta can remove them. They will gradually accumulate creating a potentially dangerous situation as cells do not function well in an acid environment. So a continuously reliable and good-quality oxygen supply is vital to the well-being of the fetus.

Viewing the placenta as a fetal lung is an extremely useful concept. The fetus cannot take air into his lungs although he is performing breathing movements, as is discussed in Chapter 6. The exchange of oxygen across the placenta is governed by all the factors that affect oxygen transfer across the maternal lung, but at the placenta there are two blood systems. The maternal uterine arteries carry blood to, and the uterine veins carry blood away from, the placenta on the maternal side. The fetal umbilical arteries carry fetal blood to and the umbilical veins carry blood away from the placenta on the fetal side. Accordingly, the factors that regulate oxygen transfer at the placenta are even more neatly regulated than in the simpler situation at the maternal lung.

Oxygen is taken up more readily by fetal red blood cells than by the mother's red blood cells because fetal red blood cells have a special form of hemoglobin. The fetal form of hemoglobin is more efficient than adult hemoglobin at catching and holding on to oxygen. This difference is another one of the little advantages that nature has provided the fetus. In addition, there is an exquisite little exchange going on in the placenta. As fetal blood goes through the placenta it sheds carbon dioxide, which diffuses to the mother across the placenta. Thus, his blood becomes less acidic and hence can take up more oxygen because of the Bohr shift. In contrast, his mother's blood is becoming more acidic as carbon dioxide diffuses into it. Accordingly, her hemoglobin releases more oxygen, thus maintaining a concentration gradient down which oxygen continues to flow to the fetus. Clever thing the placenta; it has a double Bohr shift, which doubly benefits the fetus.

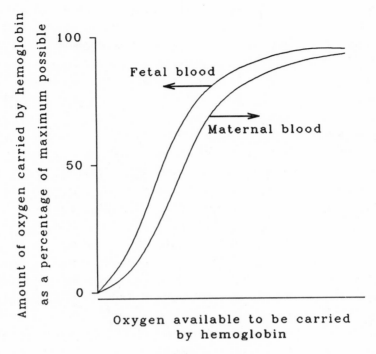

FIGURE 5.1

Oxygen dissociation curves for fetal and maternal hemoglobin. Arrows show the double Bohr shift at the placenta; fetal blood gives up carbon dioxide, so the fetus takes up more oxygen; maternal blood loses more oxygen.

No mammal can store oxygen, so in normal circumstances the fetus takes only as much oxygen from the placenta as meets his needs. He needs a mechanism to maintain his oxygen balance as he grows. Growth is a normal physiological challenge and involves constant adjustment to all his systems. As he grows he increases the amount of blood he pumps to the placenta each minute to increase oxygen uptake from the placenta. As long as the maternal and fetal blood supplies to the placenta increase in parallel with his need for oxygen, oxygen taken up will continue to match needs, and the fetus will be in balance. If for any reason the maternal circulation delivers less blood to the placenta—for example, if there is maternal arterial disease—the fetus extracts a greater percentage of the oxygen supplied to the placenta. To do this he uses several sensible stratagems. His first and immediate response is to pump more blood to the placenta. He also begins to manufacture more hemoglobin so that his total capacity to carry oxygen away from the placenta increases. This second mechanism is less rapid. It takes several days for the fetal hemoglobin to increase significantly. The systems the fetus uses to protect himself from a low oxygen supply are discussed further in Chapter 7.

In contrast to his inability to store oxygen, the fetus can store glucose as a fuel in case of a shortage coming from his mother. Glucose is stored as glycogen in the fetal heart, liver, and muscles, and in the placenta itself. Glycogen is a large string-like molecule in which hundreds of glucose molecules are joined together in a long chain. Should glucose provision to the fetus drop below his daily needs, glucose is broken off from these glycogen storage molecules and secreted into the blood for the fetus to use. However, fetal glycogen stores are small and food deprivation results within a day or so. When all his glucose stores are used up, the fetus has to break down his own precious, newly formed tissues to provide himself with energy. The problem of insufficient energy supply to the growing fetus is discussed in Chapter 10.

The last of the main functions of the placenta is as a major producer of hormones, which play important roles in the reproductive processes. Placental cells and fetal membranes synthesize hormones that are protein structures; others have a different molecular structure called steroids, which are made from fats. There is a wide variety of steroid hormones. In addition to making steroids, a major function of the placenta and fetal membranes is to alter the structure of steroids that are synthesized in other maternal and fetal tissues. The principal placental steroid hormones of interest are the estrogens and progesterone. The ability of the cells of the placenta to produce steroids, as well as to alter the structure of steroids produced elsewhere, has been demonstrated in pregnant sheep, and all primate species studied to date including women, baboons, and Rhesus monkeys.

The roles of estrogens and progesterone in maintaining pregnancy and in the processes of birth are discussed in detail in

Chapters 12 and 13. These hormones are also involved in many other cellular processes during pregnancy. An important function of estrogens is to increase blood flow in the uterus during pregnancy. As the uterus and its contents grow through pregnancy, there is a fifty-fold increase in the amount of blood flowing to the uterus. This increase in uterine blood flow is probably a result of increased production of estrogens by the placenta. Thus, the placenta very cleverly instructs the mother to increase her blood supply to the uterus so that the placenta and fetus can grow. The placenta looks after the fetus very well!

The steroid hormones produced by the mother are identical in structure to those produced in the fetus. The steroid cortisol, produced by the maternal adrenal gland, has exactly the same structure as cortisol produced by the fetal adrenal. If the fetus is to develop his own ability to regulate his cortisol secretion he must be protected against sudden bursts of secretion of cortisol by the mother. Different species use different mechanisms to protect the fetus. In sheep the placenta is relatively impermeable to cortisol. Therefore, little cortisol in the maternal circulation reaches the fetal circulation. By contrast, cortisol can cross the placenta in pregnant women and act within the fetus. However, enzymes exist within the human placenta that convert most of the cortisol that crosses the placenta to an inactive steroid and virtually cancel it out as it tries to cross the placenta.

The placenta synthesizes a wide range of hormones that have a protein structure. The best known are chorionic gonadotrophin and placental lactogen. In early pregnancy, chorionic gonado- trophin maintains the ovary's ability to secrete progesterone after the time it would normally have lost this ability had the woman not been pregnant. After ovulation, the portion of the ovary that produced the ovum, the follicle, collapses and changes its appearance and function. It becomes a yellowish structure called corpus luteum, which produces the progesterone necessary to maintain pregnancy. If the woman is not pregnant, the corpus luteum dies away after about two weeks and menstruation takes place. If the woman is pregnant, the corpus luteum must be maintained so that it can continue to produce progesterone until the placenta can take over this function adequately. Chorionic gonadotrophin from the placenta is responsible for the maintenance of the corpus luteum during these critical early weeks of pregnancy. Chorionic gonadotrophin is a hormone in the fullest sense of the word. It gets into the mother's blood, travels through the maternal blood system to the ovary, and instructs the corpus luteum to continue functioning. The extra dimension here compared with the mechanism of action of most hormones is that, in this situation in early pregnancy, we have the fetus, one organism, secreting a hormone from his cells in the placenta into another organism, his mother. The fetal hormone is then able to modify the function of cells in another organism, the mother. So the relationship between mother and fetus begins very early with a two-way conversation with the embryo already telling his mother what to do!

Placental lactogen is another important hormone produced by the placenta. In structure it is very similar to growth hormone. Many investigators feel that placental lactogen plays an important, as yet imprecisely identified, role in regulating fetal growth. It appears to act on the tissues of the mother directing them to ensure that enough food is made available to the fetus. It may also have direct effects on the growth of the fetus and placenta. Clearly, one function it has is to prepare the mother's breasts for lactation after the baby is born. While much more work is needed to establish the many roles of placental lactogen, we can see that like so many other hormones, it has multiple sites of action in the fetus, placenta, and maternal tissues.

Knowledge of the functions of the placenta and fetal membranes has greatly improved the obstetrician's ability to assess the well-being of the fetus. The major impact to date has been on diagnostic capability, being able to spot cases of placental inadequacy in good time. The obstetrician and neonatologist are then better able to make the decision whether the baby is safer maturing for a longer period of time in the uterus or whether it would be wiser to deliver the baby and look after his needs in the intensive care unit. In other words, if the fetus is not coping too well on his own, it may be wiser to shorten the period of life *before* birth to give the baby a better chance of having a life *after* birth.

For a throw-away organ we have seen that the placenta is a fascinating and complex structure. Part mother, part fetus, it has all the properties of a lung, a digestive system, a kidney, and a food store. In addition, the complexity of the hormones that the placenta produces matches all the other endocrine glands in the body put together. No wonder the Pharaohs of ancient Egypt worshipped it and carried it aloft in ceremonial processions.

Much of the work described in this chapter has been obtained by studying pregnant sheep. The sheep is one of the most efficient and useful animal models used by researchers to study both normal and abnormal pregnancy. If we are ever to understand the developmental processes that may go wrong in fetal life we must conduct at least some of the studies in the whole individual—animal or human. The test tube and the computer are very useful tools, but in the final analysis we must find out how the whole organism works. Those who would discourage research using animals often say that nothing useful is learned from such studies that can be transferred to humans. Those who have studied the history of medical research know that without research using animals we would be far less able to treat such conditions as respiratory distress in the newborn. As a result of studies in pregnant sheep we now know how steroids alter placental blood flow, how amino acids are transported from fetus to mother, and how vital hormones are secreted by placental cells into both the fetus and mother. With modifications for some differences between species, the information in this book applies to both human and animal pregnancy. We can even learn from the differences. Understanding differences between two structures or mechanisms helps us to understand each of them better, to the benefit of humans and animals.

Chapter 6

FETAL BREATHING MOVEMENTS

It is through the lungs that the gases in the air are absorbed into the body. The lungs allow exchange of oxygen and carbon dioxide between the blood and the outside atmosphere. The concentration of oxygen in the air is higher than the concentration of oxygen in the blood. Thus, there is always a tendency for oxygen to diffuse down this gradient from the high atmospheric concentration to the lower concentration in the blood. In contrast, the concentration of carbon dioxide (the waste product of cellular activities within our bodies), is higher in the blood than in the external atmosphere. Thus, carbon dioxide passes from the blood to the outside atmosphere. This exchange of gases can occur in the lungs because only a very thin membrane separates the blood in the capillaries in the lungs from the air in the air sacs of the lung.

Throughout life cells have a continuous need for oxygen. Oxygen is indispensable to the proper performance of the multitude of biochemical reactions that provide the cells with the energy required to carry out their wide range of activities. As a result of these biochemical reactions, the cells are continuously producing carbon dioxide. There is no mechanism within the body to store oxygen and only a very limited ability to allow a build-up of carbon dioxide. Carbon dioxide is an acidic compound, and when it accumulates within the body to any appreciable extent, the acidity is detrimental to the proper functioning of the body. For these reasons, the lungs must function continuously to obtain oxygen and permit the removal of carbon dioxide.

The adult lung is composed of about three hundred million small air sacs. Each air sac is about a quarter of a millimeter in diameter when fully expanded with air. The thin lining of these sacs means that there is only the smallest of diffusion barriers between the outside air in the air sac and the blood in the capillaries. The large number of air sacs provides an enormous surface area over which diffusion of oxygen and carbon dioxide can take place.

The thin layer of cells that line the lung air sacs is made up mostly of irregular-shaped cells called type I cells, which comprise most of the barrier between the air in the air sacs and the body fluids. The other lining cells are specialized cells called type II cells. The function of the type II cells is to produce a complex material that lines the air sacs and serves to reduce their surface tension. This material, called surfactant, is a mixture of very specialized lipids (the biochemical name for fats) and specialized proteins. The surface tension in any small bubble is inversely related to the size of the bubble. In other words, the smaller the bubble, the greater the surface tension in its wall. The surface tension acts to pull the walls of the bubble together and tends to make the bubble collapse. For gas exchange to occur, the air sacs must stay open. By lowering the surface tension within the air sac, surfactant plays an indispensable role in allowing the air sacs to stay expanded for the lung to function normally. The production of adequate amounts of surfactant is vital for the newborn baby to keep his air sacs open after birth and breathe air.

We will see later that cortisol produced by the fetal adrenal gland plays a key role in initiating the hormonal changes that lead to birth in sheep (Chapter 12). Cortisol infused into the fetal lamb produces premature birth. Newborn lambs born prematurely following infusion of cortisol into their circulation for two or three days are able to breathe and survive, while lambs at the same stage of development delivered by cesarean section without the previous infusion of cortisol are unable to keep open their air sacs. We now know that cortisol stimulates the activity of enzymes in the lung type II cells. These enzymes increase the production of surfactant. These findings are being put to good use in the treatment of premature babies in an attempt to increase the amount of surfactant available in the premature baby's lungs. Women at risk for premature birth are given a dose of betamethasone, a synthetic hormone with the same actions as cortisol. The betamethasone will cross the placenta and stimulate surfactant production in the fetal lungs. Then, if the baby is born prematurely, he is more likely to have enough surfactant to enable his air sacs to stay open and allow him to obtain enough oxygen. A newer form of therapy is to deliver surfactant by spraying it directly into the lungs of premature babies after birth. The surfactant used for this treatment was initially produced from the lungs of cows obtained at the slaughter house. Recently, several pharmaceutical companies have begun to produce synthetic surfactant based on the discoveries made by researchers on the composition and properties of natural surfactant. The successful development of treatment for the major problem of prematurity—immature lungs—is now saving many newborn lives that would otherwise have been lost. This is an excellent example of how basic research impacts us all.

The pulmonary artery brings blood to the lung from the right side of the heart. The blood in the pulmonary artery is the same blood that returned to the heart from the tissues of the body in the great veins. The structure of arteries is very different from that of veins. Arteries have thick muscular walls, and carry blood away from the heart. Veins are thin-walled and are the pathways by which blood returns from the tissues to the heart. In passing through the various tissues, oxygen in the circulating blood is used up, and the blood in the great veins and pulmonary artery is deoxygenated. The pulmonary artery is the only artery in the adult body that carries deoxygenated blood. From its location, coming out of the right ventricle of the heart, the pulmonary artery is clearly an artery, similar in wall structure and origin to the aorta, the large artery that leaves the left ventricle of the heart and branches into all the major arteries of the body other than the pulmonary artery.

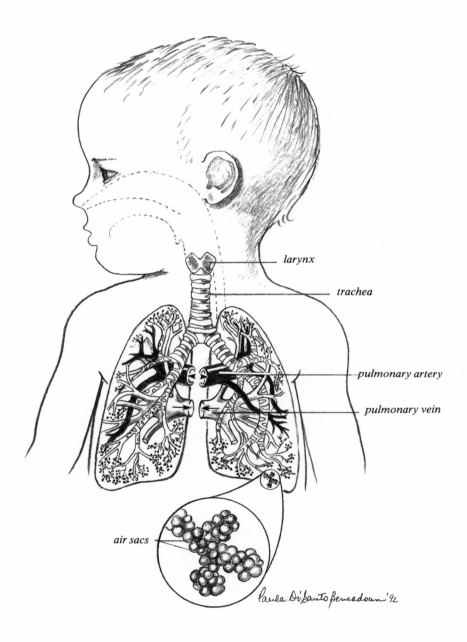

larynx

trachea

pulmonary artery

pulmonary vein

air sacs

FIGURE 6.1
Diagram of the airways from the air sacs to the outside world.

In the lung, the pulmonary artery breaks up into smaller and smaller arteries, which themselves break down into capillaries. The capillaries surround the air sacs and lie very close to their lining. Oxygen can diffuse easily from the air sacs into the blood, and carbon dioxide can diffuse from the blood into the air sacs.

The capillaries in the lung join together to form small veins, which gradually join to form the pulmonary vein. Like the other large veins in the body the pulmonary vein returns the blood to the heart. Also, like the other veins in the body the pulmonary vein is thin-walled. However, the pulmonary vein contains blood that is well-oxygenated as a result of taking up oxygen from the air sacs. It also has a low carbon dioxide content because carbon dioxide has diffused out into the air sacs. In the adult this well-oxygenated blood is returned to the left side of the heart.

Let us trace the pathway by which a single breath expels air from the air sacs to the outside atmosphere. Outlets from all the terminal air sacs join together to form small tubes that eventually join together to form one main tube on each side. These two tubes join to form the trachea. At the upper end of the trachea is the larynx. The larynx opens into the pharynx, which has several outlets, one to the mouth, one to the nose, and one to the upper part of the digestive system, the esophagus. We can trace the air pathway in reverse to follow the route that air from the outside atmosphere will take when we next breathe in: through the nose or mouth, into the larynx, and then through the trachea and eventually into the air sacs. Gas exchange will take place here. The well-oxygenated air from the atmosphere will give up some of its oxygen, and carbon dioxide will diffuse into the air in the air sac. When next we breathe out, this air, enriched with carbon dioxide, will follow the reverse route to the outside atmosphere.

The first signs of fetal lungs being formed are visible at the end of the fourth week of fetal life. A small bud now develops at the front end of the digestive tube. The digestive system is still nothing more than a primitive tube that runs the length of the fetal cell mass. The bud will form into the lungs. The bud elongates and forms the trachea and divides to form the tubes, which divide into smaller and smaller tubes until the air sacs are formed. During embryonic development, all tubes are initially formed as solid cords of cells. The airways form in the same way. It is only at twenty to twenty-four weeks of fetal development that the cords form the terminal ends of the airway passages and a lumen (central hole) is produced and they become tubes. Of course, for the duration of fetal life this lumen is filled with fluid. The timing when the lumen appears in the lung is critical. Clearly, there is no possibility that a fetus born prematurely could survive independently outside the uterus before the formation of the lumen in the bronchioles and air sacs. To survive before his lungs could be inflated with air he would need to be provided with an artificial placenta that would perform the gas transfer function of his placenta while his lungs continue to develop. Accordingly, this period (i.e., twenty to twenty-four weeks) is often perceived as the earliest moment at which the fetus could be considered a fully functional entity.

In adults the mechanical operation of the lungs is relatively simple. In order to move air into the lungs, it is necessary to create a negative pressure in the lungs with respect to the outside world. Air then moves into the lungs. If the air sacs are kept open, the air will get to the exchange surfaces close to the capillaries. The negative pressure in the chest is produced by activity of muscles of the diaphragm and chest wall. The diaphragm is a large flat muscle that stretches across the body, separating the chest from the abdomen. When the diaphragm contracts, it pulls down into the abdomen and creates a negative pressure in the chest that allows air to be drawn inward. The action of the diaphragm is assisted by the muscles of the chest wall. When we breathe in, the muscles swing the ribs upward and outward enlarging the chest, increasing the negative pressure, and allowing air to flow in from the higher pressure in the atmosphere around us.

In general, adults at rest breathe in and out about once every five seconds. Breathing out at rest is simple. When the diaphragm and inspiratory chest wall muscles relax the elastic recoil, due to the weight of the chest wall, pushes air out of the lungs. When we need to breathe more vigorously a second set of muscles in the chest wall contract to collapse the chest faster.

The nerve cells in the brain that control breathing, together called the respiratory center, are collected together in the most primitive part of our brain, the tailend of the central core that runs up and down the brain. The respiratory center coordinates the action of the breathing muscles and matches the rate of breathing to the need for oxygen. The respiratory center sends messages down the spinal cord and out through nerves from the spinal cord to regulate the activity of the inspiratory and expiratory muscles of the chest wall. These are complex control systems, able to respond rapidly to challenges such as exercise and relative lack of oxygen at high altitude. The fetus develops these respiratory control systems in the uterus, in readiness for when he is born when adequate and appropriate breathing will be vital to his existence.

Most of the information available about fetal breathing has been obtained in experimental studies in sheep carried out over the last twenty years. It is wise to ask at the outset whether data obtained from animals have any relevance to the situation in human pregnancy. It is of considerable importance to note that the same investigators who have built the framework of our knowledge of fetal breathing in sheep, particularly Dr. Geoffrey Dawes and his group at Oxford University and the late Dr. John Patrick at London, Ontario in Canada, were among the first to carry out extensive studies on human fetal breathing using ultrasound in pregnant women. These investigator-physicians noted that the great similarities between sheep and human fetuses are striking and far outweigh the differences. We can implant sensors in fetal sheep that allow us to measure and quantify fetal breathing very precisely. We can also observe and quantify the changes in breathing when the fetal sheep becomes short of oxygen, or does not have enough glucose in his blood. The same information could not be obtained directly from pregnant women. The sheep model has been responsible for showing the clinician what to look for in the human fetus.

The sheep fetus begins to make breathing movements as early as forty days of pregnancy. Pregnancy in the sheep lasts about one hundred fifty days. At this stage of fetal development, equivalent to ten weeks in human fetuses, breathing movements are virtually continuous throughout the day. Because the fetus is surrounded by amniotic fluid, he is not breathing air but is moving very small amounts of fluid in and out of his trachea. About two thirds of the way through fetal life, the breathing movements begin to occur in periods of about twenty minutes, interspersed with periods of absence of breathing. During the periods of breathing the fetus breathes at a rate of about one breath per second. The adult sheep at rest only takes one breath every five seconds.

We know that there are several factors that affect fetal breathing: some factors stimulate and others inhibit breathing movements. The proportion of the time that the fetus is breathing is determined by the balance of positive stimulation and negative inhibition to the fetal brain's respiratory center.

Fetal breathing movements can be studied in experimental animals by placing electrodes in the diaphragm and the inspiratory and expiratory muscles of the chest wall. Each time the muscle contracts, it generates an electric impulse that can be measured by the electrodes. This method of recording the contraction of muscles is called electromyography. Another innovative technique is to place small ultrasound crystals across the chest of experimental animals. One ultrasound crystal, the transmitter, is programmed to send out bursts of sound waves. The other crystal receives the sound waves. One crystal can be placed on either side of the chest. The time taken for the sound wave to pass from the transmitter crystal to the receiver crystal on the other side of the chest can be measured very accurately. The speed of the sound waves is known, so we can calculate the distance between the two crystals and obtain a continuous readout of their changing relationship to each other as the fetus breathes. In this fashion we can monitor the speed and extent of the breathing movements that the fetus makes.

Fetal breathing movements in the last third of pregnancy occur in bouts. In healthy fetuses, the amount of breathing varies with the time of day. Human fetuses have a peak in the incidence of breathing in the hours of darkness. How the fetus knows the time and what mechanisms are responsible for twenty-four-hour rhythm in the fetus are considered in more detail in Chapter 9.

We are only just beginning to understand the brain mechanisms that control the on–off periodic nature of fetal breathing. If a cut is made right across the brainstem above the level of the respiratory center in the hindbrain, then fetal breathing becomes continuous.

This shows that brain centers above the level of the section are capable of exerting an inhibitory control on the respiratory center in the fetus. If we wish, humans can voluntarily stop breathing for a short period of time. So the surprising feature in the fetus is not that breathing stops periodically, but that he stops for many minutes at a time and does so at regular intervals. In fact, he only spends about fifty percent of the time breathing. We cannot stop our breathing efforts for that long. There is another major difference between the adult and the fetus. The fetus does not need to breathe to get his oxygen. He gets oxygen across the placenta. Therefore, stopping breathing for many minutes does him no harm. Indeed, if oxygen coming across the placenta happens to be in short supply, stopping breathing does him good by saving the oxygen that would otherwise be used to make the breathing muscles work. We may wonder why he breathes at all if he does not get his oxygen through his lungs.

At the moment of birth the fetus will only have a few minutes to establish regular effective expansion and ventilation of his lungs. He will no longer have a placenta to act as his lung. In order that the newborn baby can successfully meet and overcome this urgent and vital challenge that will eventually face him, his lungs must be mature and able to produce enough surfactant. The muscle fibers of his diaphragm and all the other muscles involved in breathing must be strong and practiced. The nerve connections to the muscles from the respiratory center in the brain must be fully developed. Studies on the maturation of muscle fibers in the fetus have shown that it requires several weeks of continual activation of muscles by nerve impulses to ensure that they mature correctly. In several experimental studies it has been shown that nerve fibers play an important role in the development of the muscles.

Mammals have two different types of muscle fiber, one of which contracts slowly, and the other contracts quickly. These slow-contracting fibers are pink and contain the pigment myoglobin. Myoglobin is used to store a small amount of oxygen to allow the fibers to continue to be active during periods of oxygen lack. The other type of muscle fiber contracts very quickly. These muscle fibers are pale as they do not contain the pink myoglobin pigment.

They do not need the myoglobin because they are designed to contract extremely quickly over very short periods of time. Fast-contracting muscle fibers have activity patterns that would not benefit from a store of oxygen. By switching the nerve that should have gone to a fast muscle and directing it into a slow muscle, that slow muscle develops the appearance and behavioral pattern of a fast muscle. The reverse experiment can also be performed. Switching the nerve from a slow muscle to a muscle that normally develops as a fast muscle will change the fast muscle to a slow muscle.

These influences of nerves on muscles that change the growth and development of the muscle are good examples of cells "talking" to each other. In addition to these growth influences, muscles need to be constantly active to remain in the best shape. This need is obvious to anyone who has had a leg in a plaster cast for several weeks. When the cast is removed, the immobilized leg is very weak and the muscles look wasted, requiring exercise to get them working properly. The same considerations apply to fetal muscles including limb and respiratory muscles. So, we should not be surprised that the fetus has to practice these breathing movements while he is preparing for birth; it would be more surprising if he did not.

In addition to laying down the control pathways and developing the muscles used in breathing, fetal breathing movements have a second vital influence on the development of the fetus. Fetal breathing is essential to the normal growth of the lungs. Human fetuses that have muscle diseases that result in a decreased amount of breathing have under-developed lungs. Similar observations have been made in animals. The mechanism whereby breathing movements stimulate the growth of the fetal lung is not known. It may be due to the small amounts of fluid that move into the lung as the fetus breathes. This fluid may help to distend the lung, or may carry in growth factors from the amniotic fluid.

Having established that the fetus is performing a useful function by practicing his breathing, even though he gets no oxygen for his efforts, we can also see why the fetus is not at risk if he stops breathing for prolonged periods. He must practice, but there is no real need to breathe all day. In fact, breathing movements are tiring for the fetus. All muscle activity uses up oxygen and energy, so it is not surprising that the fetus stops breathing from time to time.

The completely undisturbed fetus breathes in periods of twenty or so minutes followed by a period of no breathing for a similar duration. There are several factors that are known to decrease the amount of fetal breathing. One of the most important of these is a fall in the amount of oxygen in the fetal blood, which is called hypoxemia. A fall in glucose in the fetal blood, called hypoglycemia, can have a similar effect. Both prescription drugs and street drugs, as well as alcohol, consumed by the mother can also reduce fetal breathing movements. Prostaglandins, which are messenger molecules produced by virtually all cells in the body, also inhibit fetal breathing.

During hypoxemia fetal breathing movements are diminished. If the hypoxemia is marked and the oxygen levels in fetal blood are very low, fetal breathing may stop completely for several hours. Adults short of oxygen, when at high altitude for example, do not stop breathing. Our response to hypoxemia is to breathe faster to obtain more oxygen from the air. The fetus, in contrast, does not get more oxygen if he makes faster breathing movements. All that happens is that he uses up more oxygen moving the muscles during breathing. Thus, it makes good sense for the fetus to stop breathing when he is hypoxemic. The cessation of breathing by the fetus in the presence of hypoxemia is called the *paradoxical fetal response to hypoxemia*. The term "paradoxical" is used because the fetal response is the opposite of the response of the adult.

A recent study by Dr. Peter Gluckman and his colleagues in New Zealand provided interesting information on the specific area of the brain that regulates the paradoxical fetal response to hypoxemia. Dr. Gluckman spent several years constructing a three-dimensional map, or atlas, of the fetal sheep brain. This atlas enables the researcher to selectively destroy very small parts of the fetal brain. Dr. Gluckman showed that a small area of the brainstem of the sheep fetus plays an indispensable role in the paradoxical fetal response to hypoxemia. When this little area of brain cells is destroyed, the fetal sheep responds to hypoxemia like an adult sheep—by increasing his rate of breathing.

As the fetus responds paradoxically, but the newborn baby responds in the normal adult fashion by increasing his breathing rate, in response to hypoxemia, some rather sudden maturation of the brain must take place at the time of birth. It appears that after birth the function of the area of the fetal brainstem that responds to hypoxemia by inhibiting breathing is either completely over-ridden or lost. The normal newborn baby will now respond to lack of oxygen by breathing faster. It has been suggested that babies who die from Sudden Infant Death Syndrome (SIDS, or crib death) may retain some function in this inhibitory brain area into newborn life. Should this happen, the baby is in a very dangerous position. If the area of the fetal brain that inhibits breathing during hypoxemia remains functional after birth, and should the newborn baby suffer from oxygen lack for any reason, such as a cold or other minor infection blocking his mouth and nose, then the inhibitory area of his brain would react as in fetal life by inhibiting breathing. The baby would accordingly become more hypoxemic, and a very dangerous, potentially fatal situation would occur, because increasing hypoxemia would only serve to depress breathing further creating a snowball effect. It is as if the newborn baby has forgotten that he is now outside the uterus and makes an inappropriate response to oxygen lack. He is trying to combat hypoxemia by using methods that were successful in decreasing his oxygen need when he was a fetus. When he was a fetus he had a placenta. Now he does not, and continuing to use fetal responses could have fatal consequences. This hypothesis is currently receiving intensive study.

When we know more about the maturation of these systems in the fetal and newborn brain, we may be able to look for markers to help us identify those babies who may still show a paradoxical response to hypoxemia after birth and are, therefore, at risk to suffer a SIDS death. Studies are being carried out to find a test to identify the babies at risk. If such a test can be developed we will be in a better position to monitor babies at risk, in our efforts to prevent SIDS. In the United States SIDS is the leading cause of mortality of infants between the ages of one and twelve months, killing between one and two of every one thousand live births. We urgently need more information if something is to be done to halt these tragic losses. Information on the maturation of these fetal and neonatal brain mechanisms requires the conduct of carefully designed experiments. They cannot be modeled on a computer without more information. Until we know what information to put into the computer there is no way we can do any modeling. There is an old saying regarding computers: If you put garbage in, you get garbage out.

Fetal breathing also decreases when there is a shortage of glucose in the fetal blood. There are areas of the fetal brain that can monitor the level of glucose in the fetal blood. If glucose levels fall the fetus responds with measures to reduce his glucose consumption, mobilize his small reserves of glucose, and initiate enzyme reactions that convert other nutrients into glucose. As glucose is his principal source of energy, stopping breathing movements, as well as other muscular movements, is a good way of conserving energy.

Fetal hypoxemia is also produced by periodic contractions of the muscle of the uterine wall. Throughout pregnancy, moderately strong contractions occur that last for quite long periods, usually between three and fifteen minutes. Some women feel them, others do not. To distinguish these movements from the strong expulsive contractions of labor, we will call them *contractures*. At the present time, although they have been seen on ultrasound videos of the uterine wall in pregnant women, we do not know how frequently contractures occur in human pregnancy. However, we know that contractures occur about once or twice an hour throughout pregnancy in sheep, cows, pigs, monkeys, and baboons. Contractures of the uterus result in a lowering of oxygen content in the fetal blood. The uterine arteries go through the wall of the uterus to reach the placenta. When the muscle fibers in the wall of the uterus contract, they squeeze the uterine arteries and reduce the amount of blood flowing through them to the placenta. The fall in uterine blood flow can be as much as thirty-five percent, with a similar fall in the amount of oxygen reaching the fetus. Experiments have been conducted to show that the fetus can sense this small fall in oxygen. It is, therefore, likely that the hypoxemia that occurs during the contracture is, in part, responsible for the cessation of fetal breathing.

In addition to the fall in oxygen content in the fetal blood during a contracture, the fetus is squeezed by the contracture. In late pregnancy, the amniotic fluid does not completely surround the fetus. The fetus is in contact with the uterine wall over large portions of his surface. Therefore when a contracture occurs, the fetus will be squeezed. We can observe and quantify the squeeze produced by a contracture by using the ultrasound-crystals technique described earlier, and continuously measure the dimensions of the fetus at several sites. The degree of squeezing exerted on the fetus not only varies with the strength of the contracture, and with the amount of amniotic fluid in the uterus, but also with the position that the fetus has most recently assumed during his periodic movements in the uterus. A contracture may decrease the front-to-back measurement of the fetal chest by over thirty percent. This is a very marked stimulus. Get someone to hug you around the chest and squeeze you so that your chest is crushed in by thirty percent, and you will see what a very considerable squeeze that is. This squeezing of the fetus will undoubtedly send a large number of nerve impulses into the fetal brain. A contracture, or squeeze, amounts to a hug for the fetus. We do not yet know exactly how contractures may modify the development of the fetal brain. However, many parts of the brain only develop correctly if they have constant stimulation and are constantly active. Perhaps the stimulation provided by contractures is part of this activity-dependent brain maturation.

At the present time it is difficult to determine which of the two stimuli, the fall in fetal oxygenation or the sensory stimulation of the squeeze, is more important in causing the fetus to stop breathing during a contracture. It is likely that both changes play a role. As will be seen in Chapter 8, contractures have several other effects on the fetus.

Recent studies have shown that prostaglandins can inhibit fetal breathing movements, and it is likely that they play a major role in the overall inhibition of fetal breathing that is responsible for the periods of non-breathing. Prostaglandins are produced locally within the fetal brain. Other fetal tissues, including the placenta, secrete prostaglandins into the fetal blood. Prostaglandin production by the placenta and fetal membranes increases in the last few days of fetal life. It is, therefore, not surprising that the amount of fetal breathing actually decreases in the last few days of pregnancy. When the umbilical cord is tied off or breaks at delivery, this source of secretion of prostaglandins into the fetal blood is lost. Suddenly, a major factor that inhibits breathing is removed. This loss of inhibition undoubtedly plays an important role in establishing continuous rhythmic breathing by the newborn.

The brain is a finely tuned machine that is very sensitive to strong chemical agents. Over-the-counter drugs, drugs prescribed by physicians, illicit drugs, and abused substances all have effects on nerve cells and/or the muscle and gland cells controlled by nerves. When a pregnant woman takes any of these groups of substances, her fetus may be affected. These agents may act either directly on the fetal brain after crossing the placenta, or they may produce effects in the fetus secondary to the changes produced in the mother. Many of these agents are able to alter fetal breathing patterns. Studies have shown that alcohol is capable of depressing fetal breathing. Alcohol will stimulate production of prostaglandins in the fetal brain, which may be the mechanism whereby alcohol inhibits fetal breathing.

Fetal breathing movements are increased when the level of carbon dioxide in the fetal blood is increased. In the adult, breathing is also increased if carbon dioxide builds up in the body. We do not know why the fetus responds similarly to the adult if carbon dioxide builds up but not when oxygen is lacking. In both of these situations the breathing efforts made by the fetus are to no avail; indeed as we have seen, they are counterproductive.

Elevated body temperatures will also stimulate fetal breathing. Temperature is clearly one of the many environmental factors that researchers have to consider closely when examining the development of the fetus.

Clearly, there are several limitations in obtaining data from human fetuses. However, the availability of ultrasound technology has enabled obstetricians to study breathing movements in the human fetus continuously for several hours. First and foremost, the obstetrician needs to know how fetal breathing patterns will change in a healthy fetus acutely or chronically exposed to specific adverse conditions. As in all branches of medicine we must understand normal function before we can properly interpret, and eventually correct, abnormal function. The obstetrician cannot put the healthy human fetus at risk by precipitating dangerous conditions. However, the obstetrician does have the opportunity to study complicated pregnancies. Even then the situation is not perfectly suitable to obtain the knowledge needed. The high-risk patient often needs rapid therapeutic action, and it is unethical to spend time just observing the fetus when treatment needs to be administered.

In addition, the high-risk patient often has several complicating problems. It is only in the carefully controlled experimental study that individual factors can be examined precisely and quantitatively. For example, we need to know the effect of hypoxemia alone on fetal breathing and at what threshold this challenge produces fetal responses and eventually brain damage to the fetus. It is important to understand the effects of hypoxemia without attendant complications of placental damage or other factors that often exist at the same time in the fetus of a difficult pregnancy. In pregnant women with placental function problems, the fetus may well be suffering from low oxygen concentrations in the blood, but the obstetrician does not know precisely the extent of the fall and how fast it has developed. Also, the obstetrician does not know what the carbon dioxide levels are and to what extent this factor is affecting the fetal response.

Correct maturation of the fetal lung and the brain's respiratory center are essential to the survival of the newborn. In the last twenty years, basic science research has used animal studies to open up a window on fetal development. The information gathered from the pregnant sheep in relation to fetal breathing movements has had an enormous impact on our knowledge of normal and abnormal function in the human fetus. All the available experimental data show that fetal breathing responses to various challenges in the human fetus have resembled the responses predicted from studies in the fetal sheep. Clearly in the fetal sheep we are in a better position to repeat studies, look at various levels of stimulus challenge, and study the different stages of pregnancy to observe any changes as the fetus matures. Individual factors can be changed one at a time in order to examine their individual effects, but this is not possible in the human.

Experiments on animals inevitably provoke controversy. There is a very strong argument for experimental studies in animals to precede investigations in pregnant women, rather than to follow them after problems and adverse side effects have been detected resulting from the use of new drugs or procedures. The greater understanding of life before birth has proved capable of saving life. By providing information to cope with problems that occur before birth, as well as with those that result from premature birth, it is increasingly likely that researchers will help us avoid distressing occurrences such as SIDS and brain damage. For those who remain unconvinced of the validity of such experimentation, it should be pointed out that animal research also provides veterinary sciences with new weapons for eliminating disease and distress in animals.

Chapter 7

FETAL CIRCULATION

We cannot kindle when we will
The fire which in the heart resides...

Matthew Arnold, *Morality*

Like little body with a mighty heart
What might'st thou do, what honor would thee do...

William Shakespeare, Chorus, *Henry V*

The heart and blood vessels are the transport waterways of the body. The heart acts as a pump that circulates the blood around these waterways. The blood leaves the heart by way of the arteries and returns to the heart in the veins. The arteries branch many times as they go into the tissues, the smallest arteries eventually leading into millions of very thin capillaries. Arteries have walls that are too thick for oxygen or glucose to leave the blood and get to the cells of the body. They are in fact sealed tubes. The exchange oi oxygen and nutrients between the blood and the cells of the body has to take place across the very thin and highly permeable walls of the capillaries. The capillaries join together to form veins, that carry the blood back to the heart completing the circuit known as the cardiovascular system.

The blood or cardiovascular system also performs a very important regulatory function as it carries hormones from the endocrine cells to the cells whose activity the hormones are designed to regulate. Furthermore, the cardiovascular system is of vital importance in the body's response to infection. Specialized cells in the blood play key roles in the body's defense against infectious organisms. Blood also carries antibodies to the site of infection to combat the invading organisms.

The overall layout of the pathways of the fetal blood circulatory system has fundamental differences from the layout of the circulation in the newborn baby and adult. The special features of the fetal circulation and the changes that must take place at birth to enable the newborn baby to maintain an independent existence outside the uterus are worth examining in some detail. We can pretend we are a small red blood cell and take a journey around the circulation of the normal newborn baby one week after birth. The red blood cell is an accomplished traveler, carrying its load of oxygen and carbon dioxide around the baby's vascular system.

The heart is like a bag of very strong muscles, with four chambers, each designated to do a job of pumping blood around the body. In the newborn circulation, as it is in adults, the venous channels returning from all over the body converge on the right atrium, or chamber. The blood in the veins has been through the various tissues of the body, which have used up most of the oxygen. The oxygen is consumed by these tissues as they go about their various tasks. Blood in the veins returning to the heart from the tissues has a rather blue color because the oxygen has been removed from the red blood cells. The hemoglobin carrier molecule in the blood cell looks red when loaded up with oxygen; when its oxygen content is low it is a dark bluish color.

When the blood arrives at the right atrium it is pumped by this muscular bag into an even stronger muscular bag, the right ventricle or chamber. The deoxygenated blood is then pumped by the right ventricle to the lungs by way of the pulmonary artery. If the lungs of the newborn baby have opened properly, the atmospheric air in the lungs contains oxygen at far higher concentrations than the oxygen in the blood that has arrived in the pulmonary artery. Accordingly, oxygen diffuses from the higher concentration in the air sacs into the blood vessels. As a result the baby's blood becomes red and well oxygenated as it passes through the lung capillaries. On the other hand, carbon dioxide, which is in high concentration in the blood arriving at the lungs, diffuses out into the air sacs. When the baby breathes out, the gas in the air sacs, including the carbon dioxide, goes out into the atmosphere. When the baby takes the next breath, air containing more oxygen enters the air sacs. Each breath is oxygen in, carbon dioxide out. It is truly awesome to consider that if a newborn baby lives to be seventy, his heart will beat one hundred thousand million times and he will take a quarter of this number of breaths. This figure seems to defy comprehension. What miraculous processes abound within our own bodies.

The newly oxygenated red-looking blood returns from the lungs in the pulmonary vein to the left side of the heart. The pulmonary vein is unique in that it is the only vein that carries well-oxygenated blood. The job of the lungs is to obtain oxygen from the air sacs for circulation to all the other tissues of the body. Once the oxygen is taken up by the blood in the pulmonary capillaries in the lungs, the blood returns to the heart. The job of the right side of the heart is to pump blood to the lungs. The job of the left side of the heart is to ensure that well-oxygenated blood arriving back in the heart from the lungs is distributed to the rest of the body.

Initially the blood returning from the lungs goes into the left atrium, which, like the right atrium, has relatively thin walls. The muscle in the wall of the left atrium pumps the blood into the much thicker-walled left ventricle. The muscle wall of the left ventricle is very thick because it has the considerable task of pumping blood all around the body. The right ventricle only has to pump the blood through the lungs. The exit from the left ventricle leads into the largest artery in the body, the aorta. This single large artery branches and branches so that the blood that initially flows through it goes to every tissue in the body, with the solitary exception of the lungs, which, as we have seen, were supplied by the pulmonary artery originating from the right ventricle and contain deoxygenated blood.

The aorta soon branches into the large arteries to the head and arms. It then curves around in the chest and descends toward the legs sending branches to all the tissues in the body wall, chest, abdomen, and legs. In animals and humans after birth, the blood going to the legs has exactly the same composition as the well-oxygenated blood going to the head and brain. It all originated in the left ventricle. The blood that has passed through and supplied the active tissues of the head with oxygen drains back to the right side of the heart in one large vein called the superior vena cava. This blood is now low in oxygen. The blood from the lower part of the body drains back in one large vein called the inferior vena cava. Venous blood in both the inferior and superior vena cava has become similarly deoxygenated. Thus in the newborn baby, with the exception of blood in the pulmonary artery and vein, all arterial blood in any part of the body has the same composition, and all venous blood in any part of the body is also uniform in composition.

If, on the other hand, we now look at the situation in the fetus, we will find that the vascular waterways are more complex. The fetus has developed some interesting and special mechanisms to deal with his particular needs and way of life while in the uterus. These are the need to oxygenate his blood using the unique and temporary organ, the placenta; and the need to give special priority to the development of the fetal brain.

The most important difference in the fetal blood system from that of the adult is that the lungs in the fetus are not used to obtain oxygen. The fetus obtains his oxygen as his blood flows through the placenta. Accordingly, the fetus has to develop special vessels to pass the blood to and from the placenta. The umbilical arteries that join the fetus to the placenta arise from the tail end of the fetal aorta and leave the fetal abdomen through the umbilical cord. The remnant of the attachment of the umbilical cord, which we call our navel or belly button, stays with us for life. From the placenta, blood returns to the body in the umbilical vein. The placenta is the site at which oxygen is picked up; consequently, the umbilical vein blood is highly oxygenated and is bright red like the pulmonary vein blood in the newborn. This well-oxygenated blood must now return to the heart to be circulated to the tissues for the cells to use in their various activities.

Blood from the umbilical vein reaches the large central vein in the lower abdomen, the inferior vena cava, which then carries the blood from the placenta back to the right side of the heart. Rather remarkably, the well-oxygenated blood in the inferior vena cava

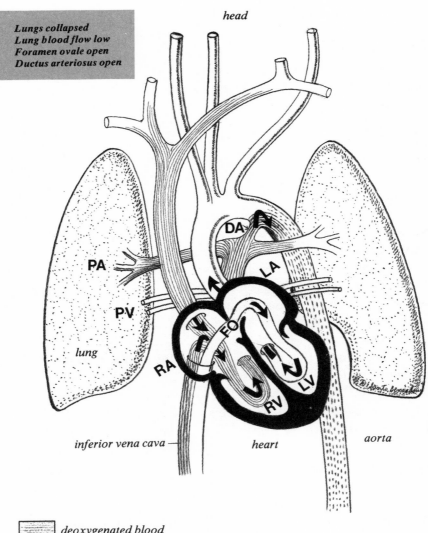

Lungs collapsed
Lung blood flow low
Foramen ovale open
Ductus arteriosus open

head

PA

PV

lung

RA

DA

LA

FO

RV

LV

inferior vena cava

heart

aorta

☐ deoxygenated blood

☐ oxygenated blood

☐ mixed blood

FIGURE 7.1

Fetal circulation. Note the two bypasses, the ductus arteriosus and foramen ovale.

RA - right atrium   FO - foramen ovale
LA - left atrium   PA - pulmonary artery
RV - right ventricle   PV - pulmonary vein
LV - left ventricle   DA - ductus arteriosus

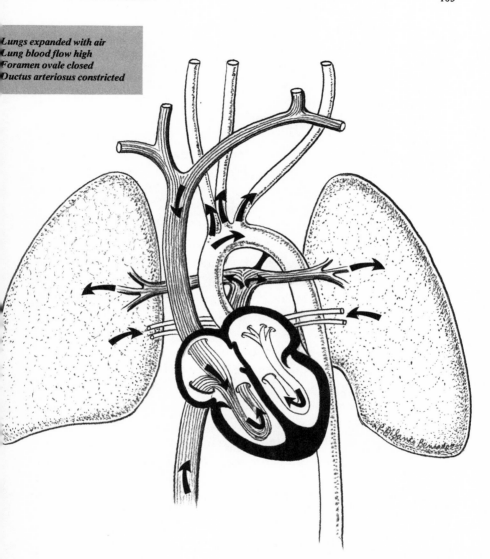

Lungs expanded with air
Lung blood flow high
Foramen ovale closed
Ductus arteriosus constricted

FIGURE 7.2

Newborn circulation. Note that the ductus arteriosus has closed and the foramen ovale flap
has shut.

from the placenta streams alongside the poorly oxygenated blood from the legs and abdominal tissues, on its way to the heart. The presence in the inferior vena cava of two streams of blood of different degrees of oxygenation is a very different situation from that in the newborn where, as described above, venous blood at all sites of the body has a very similar composition. The presence of two streams of very different blood is a direct consequence of the fact that the blood in the fetal inferior vena cava originates from two areas with very different, indeed opposite, functions. The placenta performs the function of the fetal lung; the blood returning to the heart from the placenta in the umbilical veins is well oxygenated (the red stream); the rest of the blood in the inferior vena cava is just normal venous blood returning from active tissues that have used up much of the oxygen (the blue stream). Because the blood is moving relatively slowly in the inferior vena cava and there is not much turbulence, the two streams do not mix but remain relatively well separated. This streaming is functionally extremely important.

The fetus has two bypasses, or shunts, in its circulatory system, the foramen ovale and the ductus arteriosus. These shunts separate out the streams of different blood making sure that well-oxygenated blood first goes to the fetal head to supply the developing brain, and that less well-oxygenated blood returns to the placenta to take up more oxygen. What a beautiful design feature!

The first shunt, the foramen ovale, occurs as the blood enters the right atrium. A small band of tissue diverts the well-oxygenated blood, the red stream, from the placenta across the right atrium and through a hole in the central wall of the heart that divides the right from the left atrium. This hole allows the well-oxygenated blood from the placenta to bypass the right side of the heart and the pulmonary circulation. In this way, as the lungs are not the site of oxygen exchange in the fetus, the fetus has developed a mechanism to get the well-oxygenated blood stream that is coming from the placenta straight into the left side of the heart without going through the lungs. From the left side of the heart the blood is pumped straight into the aorta. The first blood vessels that come off the aorta are the large arteries to the head, allowing this well-oxygenated blood to go straight to the head, to supply the fetal brain.

The hole in the wall that separates the right atrium and left atrium, the foramen ovale, has a flap on the left side that acts like a valve. As long as the pressure on the right side of the hole is greater than the left, the valve stays open and blood will pass from right to left. During the whole of fetal life the pressure on the right side is normally greater than that on the left. The pressure on the left side rapidly exceeds that on the right side at the time of birth, and normally the flap closes within minutes. The foramen ovale is an ingenious device that serves the fetus well for the nine months of pregnancy, but it can prove to be a point of weakness in the newborn baby. If the hole does not close, the baby will be described as having a "hole in the heart;" that is, blood will bypass the newborn baby's lungs just as it did in the fetus. In the fetus, bypassing the lungs that were not doing anything, and at the same time sending the well-oxygenated blood directly to the brain, was beneficial. However, in the newborn baby, who depends on the lungs rather than the placenta to oxygenate his blood, it is certainly not a good idea at all.

Blood returning from the fetal head and that from the lower body is by now poorly oxygenated and bluish. It passes through the right atrium into the right ventricle and then into the pulmonary artery, which is connected to the aorta by a short blood vessel called the ductus arteriosus. This is the other shunt or bypass. Like the foramen ovale, the ductus arteriosus connects the right side of the circulation, the pulmonary circulation, to the left side known as the systemic circulation. The exact site at which the ductus arteriosus joins the aorta is quite critical. The ductus arteriosus starts at the pulmonary artery and passes across to the aorta joining it at a point after where the large arterial branches go off to the head. As it is farther away from the left ventricle than the branches to the head, poorly oxygenated blood from the right ventricle and pulmonary artery will not dilute the well-oxygenated blood that was pumped across the foramen ovale through the left side of the heart into the aorta and up to the head.

The poorly oxygenated blood that passes through the ductus arteriosus into the descending aorta supplies the tissues of the abdomen and lower limbs. This blood is perfectly adequate for these slower growing tissues to develop properly. The better oxygenated blood from the placenta has been diverted to the head, and the brain will also get a better supply of nutrients such as glucose that have passed into the fetal blood at the placenta.

The direction of flow in the two shunts, the foramen ovale and the ductus arteriosus, is determined by the different pressures that exist in different parts of the circulation. Because the blood vessels in the fetal lung are constricted, and because the lung is not open and aerated, the resistance to blood flowing through the lungs is very high. In contrast, on the left or systemic side of the circulation, the placenta has widely open blood vessels and the resistance to flow is low. Blood, like any fluid, will flow down the path of least resistance. The normal direction of flow in both the foramen ovale and the ductus arteriosus during fetal life is from right to left. If the difference in resistance between the pulmonary and systemic circulations reverses, the direction of flow in the shunts also will reverse. As we shall see later, the pressure gradients reverse at birth.

The blood vessels in the lung of a newborn are very sensitive to the amount of oxygen in their vicinity. If the local oxygen levels are low, the muscle in the walls of the small arteries of the lung constrict and lower the amount of blood flowing to the poorly oxygenated part of the lung. If local concentrations of oxygen are high, the vessels open up. This responsiveness to oxygen serves the purpose in the newborn lung of taking the blood to those areas of the lung that have opened up and have a high oxygen concentration. As a result, oxygen can diffuse into the blood and be carried to the tissues. In the fetus there is no air in the air sacs, so therefore, the oxygen content in the lungs is low, and the blood vessels in the fetal lung remain tightly closed, offering a high resistance to blood flow.

In contrast to the collapsed blood vessels in the fetal lung, the small blood vessels that arise from the umbilical arteries in the placenta are wide open, so the resistance to flow in the fetal layers of the placenta is low. Because blood will flow down the path of least resistance, most of the blood in the fetal aorta goes preferentially to the placenta. In this way, the fetus' needs for obtaining oxygen and nutrients from the placenta are well fulfilled.

In the newborn, under normal conditions, blood has a more than adequate supply of oxygen and nutrients for all the tissues. Oxygen is picked up at the lung and transported to the tissues to support their need for oxygen to burn food, thereby releasing energy. Products of digestion are absorbed into the blood in the digestive system and transported to tissues where they are either put to use immediately, stored until needed, or built into the structure of the cells. Glucose can be stored in the liver and fat in fatty tissues (all too easily, more's the pity). Cells require oxygen continuously because they have no means of storing oxygen to be used in the event that the supply suddenly be cut off.

Lack of oxygen in the blood, hypoxemia, can be life-threatening. After a few seconds of pronounced oxygen deficiency, acidic compounds begin to accumulate within cells. After a few minutes, irreversible damage may occur. Cells differ in their ability to withstand periods of low oxygen and high acidity, and the cells of the brain are among the most sensitive in the entire body. Lack of oxygen for only a few minutes can lead to irreversible brain damage. The extent of the damage depends on the severity and duration of the oxygen deprivation. How much damage is caused is also determined by any past history of bouts of hypoxemia to which the fetus has been exposed.

The fetus has several ways to compensate, to maintain his well-being, during episodes of hypoxemia. In addition to stopping activities that use oxygen, such as his breathing movements, he re-directs his blood to his vital organs, the brain, the heart, and the adrenal glands, and cuts down the blood supply to the less vital areas such as the digestive system, skin, and kidneys. If the hypoxemia is severe, the muscles of the limbs cease to move so that the fetus can conserve the oxygen used in these movements. The obstetrician uses this knowledge when watching for fetal movements with the ultrasound. If there are frequent intermittent episodes of fetal movement the obstetrician feels comfortable that the baby is well-oxygenated. If limb and breathing movements are absent for prolonged periods of time, such as an hour or more, the obstetrician must consider whether the fetus is becoming compromised by oxygen lack.

Many of the functions performed by an organ in adult life are not performed by that organ in fetal life. Kidneys, for example, are vital for survival in adult life, but the placenta carries out the function of removing waste products for the fetus. Likewise, the fetus does not need his digestive system for nutrition, and does not need to move his muscles to survive. Even so, cutting down the blood supply to these and other tissues is not without risk. If the reduction in blood flow is prolonged, growth of these organs may be significantly impaired.

One special requirement that the fetus has that differs from the adult is that, however great the crisis, he must continue to get blood to the placenta in the hope that he will eventually get more oxygen from across the placenta to correct the situation. During hypoxemia of short duration, placental blood flow is maintained, and flow to the brain, heart, and adrenal glands actually increases in an attempt to maintain oxygen supply to these vital tissues. At the same time, the blood supply to the lungs, skin, muscles, kidneys, and digestive system decreases. Thus, the fetus uses two responses to compensate for oxygen lack: he decreases his activities, while at the same time re-distributing his blood preferentially to vital tissues.

Because hypoxemia causes major disturbance to normal fetal development it is very important to understand its causes. The most straightforward cause is the presence of anemia in the mother. Anemic maternal blood carries less oxygen. If insufficient oxygen is being brought to the maternal side of the placenta in the uterine arteries, delivery of oxygen to the fetus will be decreased. Another cause of fetal hypoxemia would be malfunction of the placenta. It may be damaged in some way, for example by cigarette smoking, or by cardiovascular disease in the mother. Regular prenatal care to check for these possibilities, and to treat them, is the surest way to protect the baby and give him the best possible start before life. Anemia and other potentially harmful conditions are very easily prevented or treated by good nutrition, adequate rest, avoidance of unnecessary stress, and good guidance from an obstetrician.

Many studies have been performed on the effects of both sudden and slowly developing chronic fetal hypoxemia. The results of these studies have important implications for abnormal human pregnancy, and conclusions from the animal studies are very reassuring. There is a large margin of safety built into the system. Under normal circumstances there is more oxygen delivered to the fetal tissues than is needed, and only a relatively small portion of the oxygen is extracted and used by the tissues. In times of oxygen deficiency the fetus can extract a proportionately larger amount of the oxygen in his blood, thereby maintaining his overall needs. This buffer in oxygen supply is a major defense mechanism. Experimental studies clearly show that a short-term drop in oxygen delivery for several seconds or even a few minutes does not produce damage in an otherwise healthy fetus. The fetus has developed very adequate methods to cope with a marked degree of hypoxemia, for a short period if necessary, at the time of birth.

Many erroneously believe that hypoxemia occurring during the birth process is the major cause of long-term handicap. While inadequate obstetric care or prolonged hypoxemia during delivery may sometimes cause trouble, it is much more likely that the long-term damage that leads to really harmful consequences, such as cerebral palsy, occurs as a result of several periods of hypoxemia related to some underlying conditions in the mother or the fetus occurring earlier in pregnancy. We need to improve our knowledge of fetal development so that we can decrease the incidence of fetal brain damage, prematurity, and intrauterine growth retardation.

If the lack of oxygen goes on for some time, becoming chronic in fact, the fetus produces more of his own red blood cells so that he can carry more oxygen away from the placenta. If, in spite of these defense mechanisms, the fetus still cannot obtain enough oxygen for normal growth and development, he will continue to decrease the blood flow to the less vital tissues. He continues to decrease the number of body and breathing movements, carefully conserving his decreasing energy. Oxygen and nutrients are diverted to the brain at the expense of the slower growth rate of the less vital tissues, such as muscle and some organs. In this way, the fetus may gradually become growth retarded. The growth retardation is not uniform. The growth rate of muscle and of organs such as the liver that do not perform vital roles for the fetus slows down more than the growth of the brain. We do not know precisely how these compensatory patterns of growth are brought about, but a major factor seems to be a re-distribution of the blood supply.

Decreased blood flow through an organ is brought about by powerful constriction of the blood vessels in that organ. In organs where blood flow increases, the increase is in large measure due to a decrease in the amount of constriction of the blood vessels in these areas. Two factors affect the amount of blood that flows through a tissue. One is the degree of dilation of the vessels in that tissue, the resistance to flow. The other is the general blood pressure, regulated by the amount of blood pumped by the heart. The heart can increase the amount it pumps in two ways. It can increase the rate at which it pumps, or it can increase the efficiency of each beat.

When adult humans or animals become hypoxemic they increase their heart rates to deliver more oxygen to the tissues. The increased heart rate will also increase the amount of blood going through the lungs, which assists in picking up more oxygen, provided, of course, there is oxygen available in the air. However, there is a price. The heart consumes more energy itself when it has to pump faster and stronger. The fetus adopts an opposite strategy. He maintains the amount of blood being pumped out by the heart at normal levels by increasing the force of the pumping action, while at the same time lowering the rate at which his heart beats. Thus, the hypoxemic fetus has a slower heart rate: another attempt to compensate for lack of oxygen. By shutting down the blood supply to less vital tissues, the supply to the more vital tissues can be increased without the need for an overall increase in the amount of blood pumped by the heart. So just as with the paradoxical response of fetal breathing to hypoxemia, the changes in fetal heart rate in the presence of hypoxemia are quite different from those in the adult and newly born baby. Persistence of these fetal-type cardiovascular response to hypoxemia into the newborn period may also be involved in the tragedy of SIDS.

Fetal heart rate and pattern are recorded electronically by the obstetrician because they are good indications of the overall well-being of the fetus. In both the fetus and the adult, the heart rate is regulated by nerves and circulating hormones. One set of nerve fibers increases the heart rate and another set of opposing nerve fibers acts to decrease the heart rate. By regulating the balance of activity in these two sets of nerves, the brain can very precisely control the fetal heart rate. Thus, if the obstetrician is sure that fetal heart rate patterns are normal, then this is a good indication that the parts of the brain responsible for the control of the heart rate are well oxygenated.

Circulating hormones that are released from endocrine glands at times of stress will also affect the heart rate. The most important of these hormones is adrenaline from the adrenal gland. Adrenaline will increase the rate and force of contraction of the heart muscle. Under normal circumstances the fetal heart rate is greatly influenced by all sorts of factors, such as the amount of movement the fetus is making, the amount of oxygen in the blood, and the behavioral state of the fetal brain. The normal fetus shows a continuously changing heart rate. This variability is a favorable sign that the fetus is in good health, because he is responding satisfactorily to the changes in his environment. Influences such as the change in the pressure around him, produced by uterine contractures, keep him constantly on the move, adjusting and responding, looking after himself.

With the aid of the ultrasound machine, obstetricians are now able to monitor several features of fetal heart rate and general behavioral activity, such as limb movements and fetal breathing, that previously could only be measured in experimental situations. As a result, profiles can now be composed of the overall activity of the fetus in the uterus to get an indication of his well-being. If the fetus is markedly suffering from chronic problems, early delivery by cesarean section may be needed. The fetal cardiovascular system is so well constructed that in countries where the fear of litigation is low, and the general health of women is high, the overall cesarean section rate in the whole community may be as low as two percent.

A careful study of the fetal circulatory system shows that it has small but crucial differences when compared with the adult, which are part of the subtle and ingenious adaptation to the particular situation in which he grows and develops. He has in-built defense systems to take care of most deficiencies that may arise. In late fetal life, as he prepares for life after birth, the fetus can protect himself very well in most of the difficult situations that he has to confront.

Chapter 8

BABY'S COMPUTER: THE BRAIN

*Though the Life Force supplies us with its own purpose it has no
other brains to work with than those it has painfully and
imperfectly evolved in our heads.*
George Bernard Shaw, *The Irrational Knot*, 1905

More brain, O Lord, more brain!
George Meredith, *Modern Love*

The brain is the secret weapon of the human race. It is because the
human brain is so astoundingly complex and resourceful that our
species has become the most successful one on planet earth. The
brain not only defines the human race but also the individual
within the human race. Each individual is their brain in a way
unparalleled in any other species. The lengthy period of life before
birth, and an even longer period of parental care after birth,
provides a prolonged phase of protection during which the baby's
brain undergoes a greater degree of maturation than occurs in any
other species. It is not surprising, therefore, that the brain is given
high priority in the period of growth both before and after birth.

The brain is the computer of the nervous system. To function
properly the fetal nervous system needs to develop three integrated
parts: the afferent nervous system, comprised of the input systems
required to obtain information from the surroundings; the central
processing unit, composed of the brain and spinal cord together
called the central nervous system; and the output or efferent
nervous system, the action side of the nervous system that produces
the body's responses to the environment. Together the afferent and
efferent structures are called the peripheral nervous system to
distinguish them from the central nervous system.

There are one hundred billion nerve cells in the brain of a young adult. A quarter of these nerve cells are in the most recently developed part of the brain, the cerebral cortex. This is the part of the brain that performs the most advanced activities such as rational thought and association of ideas. The brain contains another one hundred billion support cells called glial cells. The awesome and intricate web of connections between the nerve cells constitutes an immensely complicated network. During life before birth this network is gradually and systematically laid down to provide an enormous range of potential interactions between cells in different parts of the brain. Connections form between nerve cells that are close to each other as well as with nerve cells that are very far apart from one another.

The many different collections and types of nerve cells develop at different rates in the fetus. They also age very differently at the other end of their lives. Nerve cells are forming and reforming connections throughout intrauterine life. Local growth factors and hormonal regulators provide stimuli that enhance the growth of different areas of the brain at different rates at each stage of fetal development. We know that some cells only live for a short period of time; they perform their function and then die. For now, we can only guess their role. It is much more likely that these temporary cells give some short-lived yet vital instruction to other nerve or glial cells, rather than that they are just excess to the developing body's needs.

New nerve cells are constantly being "born" in all the areas of the brain. The timing of this cell birth varies in different regions of the brain. In addition to cell "birth," brain development involves programmed cell "death." All of these processes are affected by the interaction of the cell's genetic program and the body's internal and external environment.

The fetal environment is very dependent on the maternal environment and the consequences of maternal behaviors. The fetus can detect sound and perceive light; he monitors the amounts of glucose passing across the placenta from his mother, and is thereby affected by her eating patterns; he responds to changes in the uterus such as the squeezes (the fetal hugs described in Chapter 6) produced by the episodic, low amplitude contractures of the uterine muscle that occur throughout pregnancy. If his mother takes a Jacuzzi bath she gets hot; the fetus will warm up too. If she smokes a cigarette, he will indulge in some passive smoking. If she exercises more vigorously than her usual lifestyle the fetus may become short of oxygen, as the amount of blood flowing to the uterus may be reduced while she pays off her exercise-induced oxygen deficit. All of these changes will alter the amount and pattern of sensory input to the fetus. Researchers now know that the development of the brain is influenced by the degree and nature of these inputs. Brain development is dependent on activity. For example, if input from the eyes in the newborn period is abnormal, the area of the brain that processes visual information does not develop normally.

The brain is a vital personal computer. Scientists, philosophers, and theologians have constantly addressed the complex problem of the material and spiritual relationship between the "mind" and the "brain." At present there is no resolution to the issue whether there is a duality of mind and matter. It is clear that how we feel and behave are determined by the physical activities that go on at the cellular level within our brain cells. Our sensory systems by which we collect information from our surroundings, our ability to comprehend and think logically, our emotional resolution of problems, and our physical skills can all be shown to depend on efficient function of highly specialized cells within our nervous system. How often do we say, when afflicted with a bad headache, "I'm not myself?" We are acknowledging that a minor and local malfunction of the brain is impairing the total function of the personality.

As a working analog, however, the image of the brain as a personal computer is very helpful. The computer is only as good as the information that has been programmed into it. Moreover, a minor mechanical malfunction can seriously impair the machine's capacity to interpret and act upon that information.

The complex nervous system lies at the heart of personality. The nervous system develops in a miraculous fashion in the uterus. During the stages of growth and differentiation in the early embryo, specialized cells take on the three major functions of the nervous system—information gathering, central processing of the information, and taking action. We obtain sensory information through our sense organs, perform analysis and integration in the brain itself, and respond appropriately, according to the current state of activity in the brain using our nerves to control our muscles and glands. Much more is known about the development of the inputs and outputs of the fetal brain than is known about the fetal brain itself. In contrast, a great deal is known about the function of the adult brain, how it reasons and expresses emotions. The development of the brain's integrative areas is only now becoming the subject of research studies. There is much to discover about the origins of behavior and learning in the fetal brain.

The gap that exists in our knowledge about fetal brain development allows plenty of scope for moral argument. As long as we continue to know so little about the growth of behavioral and cognitive capacities we are unable to reach any conclusions about when a person becomes a person. We can say with some certainty at what point a premature baby could support an independent life, but we cannot say at what point the ingredients of personality are irreversibly assembled in the brain of the fetus. Such philosophical issues are beyond the scope of this book, and are questions for ethicists, theologians, and philosophers. Scientists can only provide the information on which to base our judgements.

Several exciting new technologies have provided methods to study the development of fetal sensory systems. Adults use five senses—hearing, vision, touch, smell, and taste. Currently, there is considerable interest in the development of the fetus' ability to hear sounds in the uterus, so let us first look at some of the features of the development of the sense of hearing.

Studies in sheep have confirmed the impression that mothers and researchers have held for a long time that sound can penetrate the uterus. These studies have provided many fascinating and important insights into fetal brain development that can be easily related to the human experience. When a loud sound is played outside the uterus an electrical discharge is picked up in the part of the fetal brain that receives sound, called the auditory cortex. This method of studying brain development is called the study of evoked potentials as the sensory stimulus, in this case sound, produces, or evokes, a potential change in the part of the brain that is responsible for processing sound information.

Researchers have found that low-frequency sound mimicking a human father's voice penetrates the abdomen and uterine wall to the fetus better than the higher frequencies of the mother's voice. Although lower frequency sounds penetrate the uterus better, the human baby can probably still recognize his mother's voice better than his father's because while he is developing in the uterus he hears her voice more often. The baby is adept at recognizing the frequencies but also the pattern of the sounds he hears in the uterus. From the sound pattern, he is able to recognize his mother's voice best of all, even immediately after birth. If his mother whispers close to one ear and his father close to the other, the newborn baby will almost invariably turn toward his mother. If the father whispers on one side and an unknown male on the other, in eighty percent of the occasions the baby will turn toward his father. Newborn babies can be shown to alter their sucking patterns if by so doing they can get a tape recorder to play their mother's voice. If the voice is in the distorted form that they would have heard in the uterus, the reaction is even stronger. These findings can be explained, at least in part, by the experiences the fetus has had during his development. They show that the fetus to some extent knows his parents before birth; this knowledge contributes to the bonding that occurs after birth.

Several groups of researchers have shown that the fetal brain response to sound is present by two thirds of the way through pregnancy. The response to a sound outside the uterus matures considerably during the last four weeks of fetal life. During this time, the electrical pattern of response in these auditory brain areas becomes increasingly like that observed in the newborn. The auditory part of the brain is not completely mature at birth, and continues to develop after birth.

Some studies suggest that newborn human babies remember tunes that they heard as a fetus. Dr. Berry Brazelton, the renowned Harvard Medical School pediatrician, tells the story of one mother who was a concert pianist. Throughout the later stages of her pregnancy she had to repeatedly practice a complicated passage from a piece she was performing. After her baby was born she did not play the piece for several months. When she did play it again for the first time, her baby was resting in his play pen. When she arrived at the complicated passage, the baby turned toward her with a quizzical look as if to say "Not again!" We do not know whether such anecdotal stories point to an ability to learn in the uterus that could be exploited to help children. Certainly there is recognition, but recognition is not learning. This research on the extent to which the fetus can perceive sound from outside his mother is still in a very early stage, and its findings have yet to be verified and assessed scientifically.

These very preliminary findings have led to exaggerated claims that fetal brain development can be accelerated or improved while the fetus is still in the uterus. As so often happens within our society, attempts to apply scientific knowledge have run ahead of the information needed to firmly establish the limits and significance of the knowledge. Dr. Thomas McDonald and I recently published a scientific paper showing that destruction of two small nuclei in the fetal brain prolonged the duration of pregnancy in sheep (see Chapter 12). Immediately these findings were reported in the national press we received many very interesting letters. Some of the letters attempted to enlist our support for small businesses who are trying to sell audio-tapes to be played to the fetus in the womb. By strapping a speaker to the maternal abdomen, these entrepreneurs claim to be able to alter fetal development. Their aim is to educate the fetus in the uterus. How these businesses thought we might help is unclear. Certainly our study involved the investigation of the fetal brain, but it only very indirectly addressed the question of fetal sensory discrimination and learning. That they did contact us, however, is an indication of how irresponsibly eager some people are to financially exploit as yet imperfectly developed scientific ideas.

There is a very real danger in taking information from scientific studies and committing the crime of Procrustes, a legendary innkeeper on the island of Cyprus at the eastern end of the Mediterranean Sea. He only had one bed in his inn. It may be that the variety of food he served and the wine in his cellar catered for all tastes, but the sole bed in the hostelry catered for only one size. Not at all daunted, he accommodated tall travelers by cutting off their legs and short travelers by stretching them. We must be careful lest we commit the scientific version of the Crime of Procrustes, which is to modify the data to suit our own preconceived notions (or business interests). It may be that one day we will know enough about the development of fetal hearing, and how sound input is hooked up to the wider aspects of brain development, to improve some aspects of fetal brain development. Until more information is available we certainly cannot tell what patterns of input may be beneficial for the fetus. Perhaps more important, we currently have no idea whether there are any harmful consequences of artificially changing the sound input to the fetus. We need much more information before parents should "put their money where their mouth is," or more precisely, where they think their baby's ear is.

There is clear evidence that the fetus can show behavioral responses to sounds. These observations have been made by using ultrasound on women as well as with experimental animal studies. What is not clear is whether these responses result in favorable changes in the development of the fetal brain and fetal behavior. Some studies have shown that the way the fetus responds to a sound source placed on the abdomen suggests that he has been startled. Being startled may not be disadvantageous to the fetus. There is evidence that newborn rats that have been handled at a young age are less stressed in strange situations when they are fully grown. It may be that if we have experiences that "tone-up" our response systems while we are developing, such experiences leave us better prepared to deal with stressful situations later.

If the fetus is exposed to a particular sound repeatedly, he eventually adapts and ignores it. The behavioral psychologists call this adaptation, or habituation. Fetal habituation to sound can be seen if we observe a human baby on the ultrasound machine. If we place a buzzer on his mother's abdomen and play a sound, the fetus moves. He is responding to the sound. If we repeat the sound every thirty seconds, after the fourth or fifth repetition of the sound, the fetus no longer responds to the sound. He habituates. There is also evidence that a very pronounced sound stimulus to the fetus modifies future responses to sound.

Light penetrates the abdominal wall and may under certain conditions alter fetal function. By placing a bright light source on the mother's abdomen and flashing it on briefly we can demonstrate that the fetus moves his head toward the light source. Again, repeated flashes lead to habituation; the fetus ignores the repeated flash of light—it is no longer novel for him. Hormone concentrations in fetal blood differ at different times of the year and there is evidence that some of the differences are due to the direct effects of light on the fetus. Other effects of light probably occur indirectly as a result of changes in the mother produced by daylight and darkness. Several aspects of how environmental and maternal rhythms affect the fetus are discussed in the next chapter. As mentioned before, we do know that input from the eyes in the newborn will influence the development of the parts of the brain that process visual information. We need to know much more about the extent that maturation of the fetal brain is influenced by activity and environment.

In our present state of knowledge it is impossible to say whether sound or any other form of sensory stimulation of the fetus is beneficial or harmful. Indeed it is currently impossible to state whether the effects of any form of fetal stimulation are lasting, although the available evidence does suggest that some effects last at least a short time. "If in doubt, leave it out," or as Voltaire put it "In ignorance abstain," is a good course to follow in the interest of safety. At present we are still fairly ignorant, so now is not the time to bombard the fetus with external sounds or flashing lights. Unfortunately, too often economic imperatives or entrenched philosophical or doctrinal positions attempt to preempt the ground that should be left to the accumulation of facts rather than opinions, forcing the pace unnaturally and reaching conclusions without mature deliberation.

Another excellent example of activity-dependent development is the maturation of the area of the cerebral cortex that receives information from the whiskers on the noses of mice. Mice are exquisitely sensitive to information obtained from their whiskers. The nerve fibers that run from the whiskers pass through a series of interconnected nerve cells and carry the information to a particular area of the cerebral cortex. This area of the brain has nerve cells arranged in barrel-shaped clusters. Each barrel corresponds to a whisker. If a single whisker is removed from the mouse at the time of birth, the barrels that correspond to that whisker do not develop. As mentioned earlier, similar studies have shown that removing the visual input from the eyes alters the development of the part of the brain that analyzes visual information. Without adequate and appropriate sensory input the central nervous system cannot develop correctly. Similar consequences of activity-dependent maturation have been shown in newborn rats, which, when maintained in a bland and featureless environment, display retarded exploratory and learning skills. Like a muscle, the brain needs exercise. Without correct development of the central nervous system, behavioral integration will be altered. Behavior is essentially the final expression of the sorting of all our sensory input, and the central processing of that information to allow us to interact with our environment. Behavior is the active expression of personality.

Of course, a fundamental element of personality is gender. At what stage and in what way sexual differentiation affects the development of the brain is an important study in itself. Few topics raise the temperature of social discussion as much as the existence and nature of gender differences. At birth, the outward differentiation of the two sexes is usually very clear. In Chapter 4 we saw that paracrine regulators and hormones from the male gonad, the testis, imposes the male developmental program on the reproductive tract.

The same basic rule of sexual differentiation operates for some of the major gender-related differences in the structure of the brain. Several studies pioneered at the Netherlands Central Institute for Brain Research under the leadership of Dr. Dick Swaab, and also by the research group at the University of California, Los Angeles under Dr. Roger Gorski, have shown that collections of nerve cells in the hypothalamus are much larger in the male than in the female. Of course, size is not everything. These nuclei in the hypothalamus are called the sexually dimorphic nuclei. They are called dimorphic because they can be two shapes: one shape in females and another in males.

Sexual differentiation of reproductive behavior patterns is controlled by the brain. An ovary transplanted successfully from a female to a male rat continues to secrete female estrogens, but the rhythmic pattern of estrogen secretion that corresponds to the ovarian cycle of the female rat is lost. From this observation we know that the rhythmic cycles of the female require the presence of more than the ovary. A pituitary gland successfully transplanted from a male to a female rat maintains the normal function of the ovaries of the female. The rhythmic pattern is maintained by the male pituitary. Accordingly, we may conclude that the rhythmicity of the female reproductive cycle resides in the brain. These observations point to the hypothalamus as the control center. The hypothalamus is known to control the rhythm of reproductive hormone secretion in adults.

In the early 1960s Geoffrey Harris at Oxford University performed an experiment that went a long way to explaining the whole process of sexual differentiation of the brain. He injected newborn female rats with the male sex hormone, testosterone. When he gave just a single injection on the first day of newborn life, nothing happened immediately to the newborn females. As they approached puberty, the ovaries of these testosterone-treated female rat pups seemed to develop normally. The ovaries formed follicles and appeared to grow normally for the forty days or so before puberty. However, when female rats that had received just one injection of testosterone on the day after birth eventually came to puberty, they did not release their pituitary hormones in a rhythmic cycle. Their ovaries looked just like mature ovaries transplanted to an adult male rat; they could function normally in every respect except that they did not cycle. If Harris gave the single injection of testosterone to newborn female rats after the fifth day of newborn life, there was no long-term effect. When these female rats reached puberty they started normal ovarian cycles.

Harris' experiments in the rat show that at a critical stage in brain development of only two or three days duration, if male hormones are present, the brain is conditioned once-and-for-all not to produce the normal rhythmic secretion of the brain and pituitary hormones that regulate the rhythms of female reproductive life. As a result, the brain will function as a male throughout the whole of the animal's life, although the rat's genetic makeup is female. Microscopically, if we look at the sexually dimorphic nuclei in the hypothalamus of the genetic females that were made acyclic by testosterone injections, the nuclei are indistinguishable from the male form. The testosterone has acted at a critical period of development to program this regulatory part of the developing brain to remain permanently acyclic. In the rat, the critical period at which these sexually dimorphic brain structures differentiate occurs after birth. In the human and many other species, these same critical phases occur before birth.

Studies such as those conducted by Harris show that there are firm biological bases for sexual differences in behavior. There is in every animal, including humans, a genetic program that determines either male or female sexual behavior. This program can be tampered with by the use of drugs or it can be adjusted by nurture, education, and environmental factors in the course of life both before and after birth. The fundamental difference between male and female remains a biological phenomenon that is etched into the genetic structure. The final outcome will be a summation of the influence of the genetic program and the internal and external environment.

The development of the brain, and the central functions of the nervous system, remain one of the last frontiers of neuroscience and biology. The National Institutes of Health have labeled the 1990s the "Decade of the Brain." We will undoubtedly learn more about the development of the fetal brain. This information will be enormously exciting and also have great practical use. With firm, scientifically based information we will at last be able to do something to anticipate, prevent, and treat such lifetime disorders as autism and cerebral palsy. The obstetrician will have a better handle on why brain damage occurs in some fetuses exposed to minimal challenges, and the reasons why others far more seriously stressed are unaffected.

Each wrinkling of a newborn baby's face tells a little of what is going on in the baby's brain. Dr. Brazelton has pioneered ideas on the ways newborn babies try to control their behavioral responses. His behavioral assessment scale for the newborn has been adopted worldwide for the evaluation of newborn development in human babies. He has shown us that the brain has a "cost of doing work." It appears that the newborn baby needs to spend time at different levels of sleep, just as much as he needs to spend time receiving input from and exploring the environment. At times the newborn baby appears to be actively trying to go to sleep and to re-organize his brain activity. At such times it is best to help the baby achieve his goals rather than disturb him for some reason or other. This information on behavioral development of the newborn will help researchers to design studies for the much more difficult task of evaluating the fetus' behavioral development. As we learn more about the development of the fetal brain and fetal behaviors we will be better placed to help the fetus through his critical periods of fetal brain development and the transition from the uterine to the external environment. This ability to help the fetus may be of considerable importance in unfavorable situations such as growth retardation.

If there were a Brazelton behavioral assessment scale for the fetus we could chart developmental problems before birth. We would be able to identify the fetus who is not going through the correct sequence of intrauterine developmental stages, and help the parents to take corrective action: to avoid stressful situations, to eat better, or change their lifestyles. The ultrasound machine has provided parents with a window by which they can learn about their baby, understand how his movements change, and prepare for his joyous arrival in the outside world. It can also help us to provide him with his needs during development.

Behavior, being the outward manifestation of what is going on inside the brain, is at present easier to examine than the inner workings of the brain. This is especially true in the fetus, and research scientists must of necessity concentrate their attention on this outward expression of brain function. Behavioral scientists use special investigational tools to look at the underlying mechanisms that are related to differences in our behavior. Researchers are interested in the factors arising within the brain as well as those from the environment outside the brain that determine our behavior. To evaluate these factors that regulate behavior the researcher needs to undertake detailed observation of different behavioral states under a full range of different situations. The most commonly used readouts of behavioral state changes are patterns of breathing movements, as observed in Chapter 6, eye movements, brain waves, body movements, and heart rate, which change as a result of the output from the brain, as seen in Chapter 7. Specific patterns of these different features occur in different states. The best example of these differences are those that occur during sleep.

By placing electrodes on fetal sheep in the uterus, and studying development of the fetal brain-waves over several days, we know that the fetus has bouts of sleep and wakefulness. Rapid eye movements (REM) occur during some of the time the fetus is sleeping. During REM sleep the brain-wave pattern shows small, irregular, and very rapid spikes. This pattern of sleep is similar to REM sleep seen when adults dream. It is sometimes called active sleep. Of course, we do not know whether the fetus is really dreaming and, if he is, we have no information about the content of these dreams. It is unlikely that any fetal dreaming is similar to our dreams. Dreams are based on experience. We can only dream on a "full mind." The other type of sleep pattern observed when we record from the fetus is called quiet sleep, or slow wave sleep, because the brain-wave record shows very characteristic large, regular slowly recurring spikes. Each of these recorded brain-wave activities is matched by specific recorded eye movements (or lack of them), and patterns in limb movements, heart rate variability, and breathing movements.

Physicians and researchers who study behavior look for stable patterns in which several behavioral features occur together. In the 1960s and 1970s pediatricians began studying premature babies to observe the level of development they attained before birth. It soon became clear that very premature babies born after only twenty-four to twenty-seven weeks of pregnancy remained constantly in

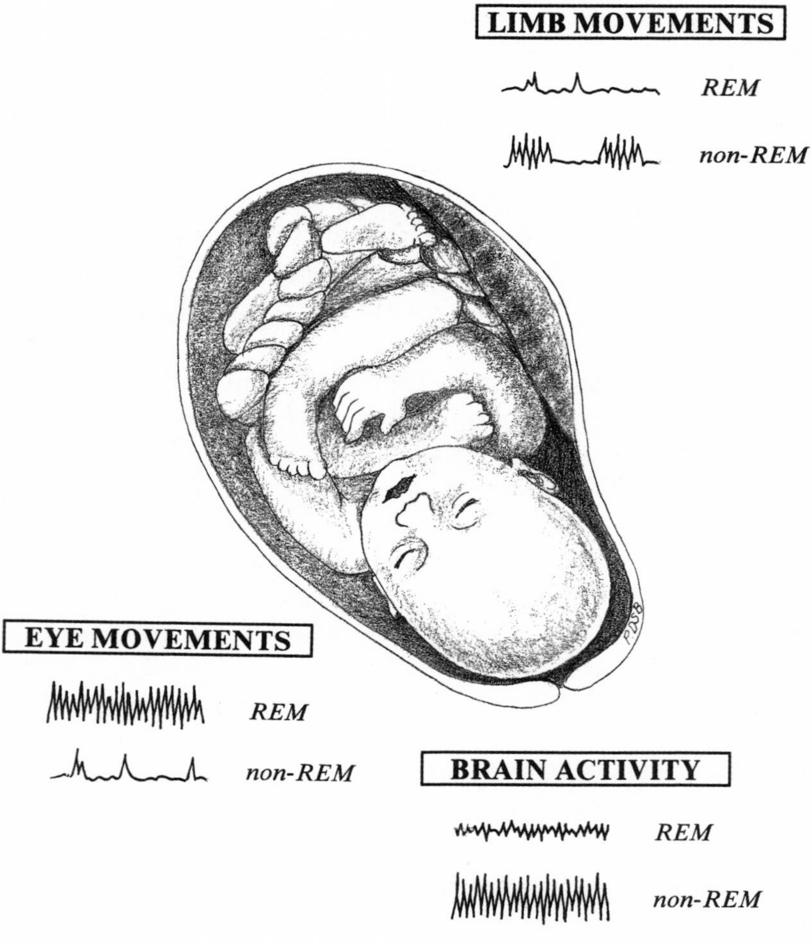

FIGURE 8.1

In the final weeks of life before birth the fetus is switching through different sleep states. Recordings of eye movements, movements of the limbs, and fetal breathing show different behavioral patterns at different times. These behavioral states are controlled by the fetal brain.

only one unchanging behavioral pattern, which could not be characterized as sleep or wakefulness by the usual criteria. When premature babies were studied in the nursery, at the equivalent of thirty-two weeks of pregnancy, two different patterns of brain activity began to emerge. However, it was not until the equivalent of thirty-seven weeks of pregnancy that active and quiet sleep could be clearly distinguished.

These findings have been compared with observations made on the human fetus in the uterus by means of the ultrasound machine. This approach has provided fascinating insights into the development of human fetal behavior patterns. We now know that the fetal behavior patterns develop in the uterus in a manner very similar to their development in premature babies. We can now see with the aid of ultrasound how the fetus alters his breathing patterns, movements, and reactions in response to alterations in his intrauterine environment.

After thirty-two weeks of pregnancy, clear and well coordinated fetal behavioral states begin to emerge. The time spent in each of these states, and the ease with which the fetus moves from one to the next, can tell us much about the maturation of the fetal brain, and its ability to receive information and to respond to it. Ultrasound studies have shown that fetal behaviors can be altered by certain abnormal developmental conditions. For example, growth retarded fetuses spend less time breathing and moving. This decreased energy expenditure by the fetus probably represents an attempt to compensate for the lack of oxygen and nutrients that have led to the growth retardation. However, we need to ask ourselves, "What are the long-term consequences to the fetus of this decreased amount of movement?" Remember, much fetal brain development depends on activity in order to occur properly: it is activity-dependent. We need to know what are the consequences of a decreased amount of movement to the normal development of fetal brain and limb muscles. We do know that fetal lung development is impaired when fetal breathing movements are markedly diminished.

Simultaneous activity of different parts of the brain is expressed as a behavior pattern. One of the most striking patterns is the day/night, rest/activity, or sleep/wakefulness pattern. In the next chapter we will see that certain areas of the brain have their own built-in rhythms that return approximately every twenty-four hours. This rhythm can be set to different time lengths by regularly repeating external stimuli. The most important of these external timers is light, which programs most animals to the day/night or light/dark rhythm.

Differing patterns of brain activity at different times of the twenty-four-hour day are clearly important to mammals for many of their activities: to the predator in determining when to hunt; to the prey in avoiding the predator; and for reproduction in bringing male and female together at the optimal time of the reproductive cycle. This inherent periodicity in brain function must begin to manifest itself at some identifiable stage of development. Considerable evidence is accumulating to show that twenty-four-hour rhythms can be observed even in the fetus. Whether these rhythms are intrinsic to the fetus or are driven by maternal factors needs careful consideration of the evidence in each case. This fascinating topic is further explored in the next chapter.

The fetus has been observed to do a lot of swallowing, which helps to regulate the amount of fluid in the amniotic cavity. The passage of amniotic fluid into the fetal digestive system is necessary for normal growth and development of the digestive system because amniotic fluid contains growth factors that help the digestive system to grow. Swallowing by the fetus is the major way the volume of the amniotic cavity is regulated. If the fetus stops swallowing for any reason, a condition known as polyhydramnios (too much fluid in the amniotic cavity) occurs. Polyhydramnios can be a dangerous sign that the fetal brain is not functioning normally to produce the correct amount of swallowing activity. It can lead to premature birth by stretching the muscle in the uterine wall, thereby stimulating it to contract.

Fetal breathing is another observable behavior pattern. We saw in Chapter 6 that the fetus breathes episodically and that the number and length of episodes were decreased by hypoxemia. This unexpected response is the fetal paradoxical response to oxygen lack. The regulatory role of the fetal brain in controlling fetal breathing and fetal movements is currently the subject of considerable study.

A profile of all the observable fetal movements throughout the day is the best readout that the obstetrician has that the fetal brain is developing normally and is not under any short- or long-term stress. The obstetrician will look at the fetus with ultrasound for at least twenty minutes and note the amount and quality of fetal limb movements, fetal breathing movements, the fetal heart rate, and the amount of amniotic fluid. Analyzing the composite pattern of all these features, the obstetrician can compose a biophysical profile of the fetus. The amount of amniotic fluid appears to be particularly important. When the fetal brain is stressed it releases antidiuretic hormone. The name "antidiuretic hormone" describes the hormone's ability to decrease the amount of urine the fetus produces. Because the urine is the major component of the amniotic fluid, a decrease in urine production by the fetus will lead to a decrease in the amount of amniotic fluid. Measuring the amount of amniotic fluid seen on the ultrasound picture is a good overall index of the amount of antidiuretic hormone the fetus has secreted, which gives an indication of the degree of distress the fetus has been under in the last day or so.

We have seen that the periodic bouts of activity of the uterine muscle, contractures, occur throughout pregnancy in sheep and other animals. These contractures are an important source of input to the fetal nervous system. One of the things they do is to cause the fetus to stop breathing. They also tend to change the sleep state of the fetus. If the fetus is in REM sleep and a contracture occurs, the fetus is very likely to switch out of REM sleep. The periodic contracture activity changes the fetal environment in several ways. As the muscle of the uterine wall contracts it squeezes the blood vessels that are passing through it to the placenta, thereby decreasing the blood flow. As a result of this fall in uterine blood flow, less oxygen gets across to the fetus. The decrease in the amount of oxygen in the fetal blood is small, too small to be a life-threatening risk to the fetus providing he is otherwise healthy. However, studies show that the fetus can perceive this small fall in oxygen and respond accordingly by stopping breathing and secreting several hormones, which mobilize the body's response to stress.

We have seen that when a contracture occurs, the fetus is squeezed. Sometimes the fetal chest decreases its front-to-back measurement by as much as a third, constituting a pronounced stimulus to the fetus. In addition to lowering the amount of oxygen in fetal blood and producing a squeezing stimulus to the fetus, contractures will raise the pressure in the fetal head. All of these stimuli will combine to change the fetal environment, and probably play a very important role in stimulating formation of nerve-cell connections in the brain.

A less-than-welcome source of stimuli to the fetal nervous system are drugs taken by his mother. Drugs-of-abuse have marked and long-lasting effects on the developing fetal brain. The most striking, and best studied, example is cocaine, which markedly disorganizes the normal relationships of the different components used to study behavior such as breathing and body movements. Cocaine interferes with the regular pattern of behavioral states and the transitions from one state to another. The problem of drug, tobacco, and alcohol abuse and how they affect fetal behavior and brain development is discussed in more detail in Chapter 11. It is relevant at this point to note that drugs-of-abuse can seriously affect the fetal brain. In one study, mothers were tested at a time when their urine proved positive for cocaine and tested again within a week when their urine was negative. When the mother was positive for cocaine the heart rate pattern in the fetus was very different from the pattern observed when the mother was free of cocaine.

There are short- and long-term benefits that will accrue from more knowledge and a better understanding of fetal brain development. Inevitably, the baby is not developing in an environment that is constant. During the day the mother is moving around, eating at various times, and altering the amount of noise and other stimuli to which she is exposed in the environment around her. The ability of the fetus to respond to these changes is used by the obstetrician as an index of normal development. The obstetrician can record the fetal heart rate continuously from the mother's abdomen using ultrasonic techniques. The heart rate can be shown to change throughout the day. The most pronounced

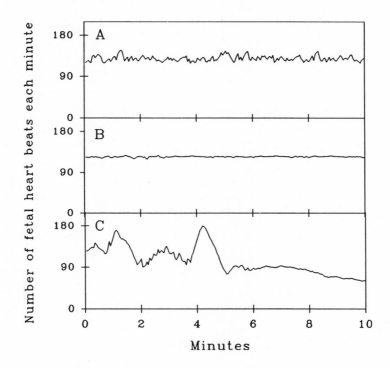

FIGURE 8.2

Fetal heart rate patterns. (A) Normal fetal heart rate variability is seen in the well-oxygenated fetus. The brain sends changing instructions to the fetal heart to keep the rate going up and down periodically as shown by the peaks and troughs. (B) No fetal heart rate variability. The brain does not send continuous changing instructions to control fetal heart rate, which is flat and constant. Further tests are needed to determine whether the fetus is short of oxygen. (C) Sudden slowing and loss of heart rate variability. This dramatic fall and loss of peaks and troughs indicates that the fetus is short of oxygen and something probably needs to be done soon to deliver the baby.

normal changes are the accelerations of the fetal heart rate associated with fetal movements. These suggest a healthy fetus.

In a test of fetal well-being used during a woman's pregnancy the obstetrician observes the normal spontaneous variation of fetal heart rate. This test is called the non-stress test because no specific challenge or stress is provided to the fetus or mother; the obstetrician just observes the spontaneous changes. The oxygen-deprived fetus does not show spontaneous periodic fluctuations. If the obstetrician is concerned about the fetus' ability to respond to his environment, there are two very good ways of stimulating the fetus to see if he can respond, one being a fetal stimulation in which a vibrator is placed on the maternal abdomen to cause a change in fetal heart rate. The other is the oxytocin stress test, in which a small amount of oxytocin is administered into a vein of the mother to make her uterus contract. This will stimulate the fetus, and the heart rate response is evaluated. In each of these tests the obstetrician is looking for indications that the fetal brain is able to collect information, process it, and send out appropriate signals through the nerves to control the rate at which the heart beats. In the short term a better understanding of how the fetal brain develops will enable the obstetrician to devise other equally illuminating tests that will improve the management of problem pregnancies.

Several long-term benefits will also accrue. Every year in the United States, eight thousand babies die of Sudden Infant Death Syndrome (SIDS) within the first year of life. These babies clearly have abnormal respiratory and heart rate responses. In essence they behave inappropriately under certain life-threatening situations. Many studies have shown that babies who die of SIDS have abnormalities in their breathing responses to lack of oxygen. Abnormalities can often be observed in their brothers and sisters and even their parents. We desperately need information that tells us why the brains of these unfortunate babies appear not to have matured to the point where they have the ability to make the appropriate responses to changing environments. There is much to learn about the effects of prenatal stressors and other types of experiences on brain and behavioral development.

Many of the studies on early brain and behavioral development have been conducted in newborn rats, because the rat is born at a stage when his brain is very immature compared with the brain of human babies. Those phases of brain development that occur before birth in the human baby and are more difficult to study, occur after birth in the rat and can, therefore, be more easily studied. Several studies have shown that fetal or newborn rats exposed to stressors of various types will respond differently to stress in later life when compared with rats not exposed to the stressor. In some instances just injecting the fetal or newborn rat with the adrenal steroids they release in times of stress will have the same effect as early exposure to stress on responses later in life. We have already seen that testosterone, also a steroid, plays a profound role in organizing the sexual differentiation of the brain. By the same token it should not be so surprising that related steroids produced by stress in the fetus can also have permanent effects on the developing brain. There is much to learn about the effects of prenatal stressors and other types of experience on brain and behavioral development.

Throughout this book we have seen how the fetal genetic program unfolds while interacting with the environment, both immediate and distant. The correct alignment and interaction of the two hundred billion cells in the nervous system is brought about by an awesome series of developmental events involving cell division, cell migration, cell interaction, and cell death. This same genetic program provides for the development of a system as complex as any cosmic array of stars or galaxies. It is no wonder that we are all different in how we think and how we react to our environment. Even identical twins are not exposed to exactly the same intrauterine influences. One of them is bound to have a better blood supply than the other. Understanding the way differences in brain function arise during life before birth, and preparing the way for development after birth, are exciting challenges for medical science. With every passing day research into fetal brain development improves the chances that every baby can enjoy its fundamental birthright—a healthy brain—so necessary for human happiness and a fulfilling life.

Chapter 9

FETAL RHYTHMS

Perfection is the Child of Time.

Bishop Hall

Ev'ry member of the force, Has a watch and chain, of course; If you want to know the time, Ask a p'liceman!
E.W. Rogers, Edwardian Music Hall Song

That period of twenty-four hours, formed by the regular revolution of our earth, in which all its inhabitants partake, is particularly distinguished in the physical economy of man...It is, as it were, the unity of our natural chronology.
C.W. Hufeland, *The Art of Prolonging Life.*
Second English translation, London 1797

Whether we worship it or not, we are all ruled by the sun. Each day the approximately twenty-four-hour rhythm of the earth's movement around the sun imposes itself on the patterns of our lives. It is vital for animals to be adjusted to live by this solar rhythm. Arriving at the watering hole too early or too late may mean that a water buffalo will encounter predators that would not be there at other times of the day. While such primitive dangers do not generally beset humans any more, we are still endowed with a body clock that has the ability to anticipate events that occur at the same time each day. We do this by adjusting all our bodily functions to the solar day.

Scientists interested in biological rhythms have shown that there is a "clock" (the hypothalamus) in the human brain that helps us to organize ourselves. From the evolutionary point of view this is a very old part of the brain. A small group of nerve cells within the hypothalamus (the suprachiasmatic nucleus, or SCN for short), has an intrinsic rhythm of activity. If some of these cells are put in a dish surrounded by a solution containing essential nutrients, the nerve cells exhibit a pattern of cyclical activity, approximately twenty-four hours long.

Cycles that repeat themselves approximately every twenty-four hours are known as circadian rhythms. This name is derived from two Latin words, "circa," meaning "about" and "dia," meaning "a day." At first sight it may seem surprising that the activity of the nerve cells in the clock is not exactly twenty-four hours, but in fact on only two days each year is the day/night cycle exactly twenty-four hours long. If the clock in our brain were locked to exactly twenty-four hours it would be more often wrong than right. Locked to twenty-four hours it would be in conflict with the changing information we obtain from the world outside us. So, the clock has the flexibility to allow for small daily adjustments to keep in synchrony with the changes in light and darkness that govern our daily rhythms. The way the light/dark rhythm of the environment sets the SCN clock is called entrainment. In so doing, it keeps our clock in line with the continuous and gradual change in the length of day.

In the early days of research in this area, people believed that our twnety-four-hour rhythms were simply the result of the environmental cycle. We now know that if all outside cues are removed, the SCN clock will continue to function with its own rhythm. Studies to investigate the characteristics of the intrinsic rhythm of the clock have been conducted in animal experiments, as well as in people who have gone into deep caves or isolated rooms, without any information relating to time in the real world outside. In these situations the changing daylight and other potential entraining cues such as meal times are removed. During this type of isolation, individuals gradually lose their synchronization with the world outside. Circadian rhythms in animals who are active by day seem to have a clock that counts a day as less than twenty-four hours, and night-active animals have a clock with a cycle slightly longer than twenty-four hours. Each of us has a slightly different clock. Two people isolated from each other in separate rooms would probably end up on completely different time schedules.

Jet lag occurs when there is a mismatch between our own internal time (the time to which our SCN clock is set) and the time in the world outside as perceived by the brain. If I fly overnight from New York to London, England, I arrive at Heathrow in

London at seven in the morning. My brain observes what is going on around me. The London rush-hour is just starting; people are having their breakfast. I can immediately set my watch to the London time. It is not so easy for my internal time-keeping system to reset itself. My SCN clock is still functioning on New York time, telling my brain and the rest of my body that it is only two o'clock in the morning. The light outside is contradicting this internal information. My body becomes confused and I must adjust. This adjustment takes a few days. In most people it takes one day adjustment time for each hour of time difference. During the few days of adjustment, the brain is registering the new information coming in from the external light and dark cues, meal times, and the activities of the world around me. It then passes this information to the SCN clock, which resets the different rhythms of the body to match the new environmental cycle. During this period of adjustment internal confusion reigns because some internal rhythms may adjust faster than others. The period of jet lag continues until all rhythms are back in synchrony. It can be a very confusing experience for the brain.

The fetus appears to be able to tell the time. Many of his bodily functions demonstrate a twenty-four-hour rhythm, such as his heart rate and his breathing movements. We need to know whether these fetal rhythms are driven by the fetal SCN or whether they are simply the result of passive responses to rhythms in the mother.

We know that some hormones can pass from the mother to the fetus across the placenta. It is possible that the rhythms in the fetus are just the response of the fetal heart and brain to these transplacental signals. We must be careful to separate the two issues. First, we need to know whether the fetal SCN is functioning while the fetus is in the uterus. If so, we also need to know if and how the fetal SCN receives its day/night information from his mother. In other words, we must find out whether the mother entrains the fetus to her twenty-four-hour rhythms. If she does play a role in getting him into synchrony with her own rhythms it will prove useful for the fetus who, as a result, will be prepared to enter the same world in which she lives.

Studies conducted in rats do suggest that the fetal SCN clock is functioning in the uterus. It is likely that the SCN is functioning at birth in species like the human that are born in a fairly mature state. It is not just an academic question as to whether the SCN in the newborn has its own independent rhythm. The newborn baby must adjust to his environment; he needs to have a functioning time-keeping system in his brain in order to function in the context of the twenty-four-hour day.

As we have seen, even if the fetus has a functioning SCN clock, he needs precise information about the outside world in order to adjust his circadian clock (which you will remember is not exactly twenty-four hours). Information about the day/night rhythm of the outside world passes from mother to fetus in many ways. As the mother eats her meals, her blood glucose rises for a few hours after each meal. The magnitude of the increase will depend on the size of the meal. The increase in the concentration gradient of glucose from the mother to the fetus across the placenta results in an increase in the passage of glucose to the fetus and a rise in the concentration of glucose in the blood of the fetus.

It is very possible that the fetus can use the changes in the levels of glucose and other molecules in his blood as cues to the time in the outside world. We know that the fetus can respond to some of these maternal messages. The hormone cortisol has been shown to cross the placenta in the monkey. When there is a build-up in the concentration of cortisol in the fetal blood that has crossed from his mother, the fetus switches off his own cortisol production. In this way he can monitor these changes. It just so happens that the nerve cells in the SCN have receptors on their surface for cortisol. Thus, one mechanism by which the fetus would be informed what time it is in his mother's world is the amount of cortisol that has come across the placenta from his mother's blood. In this way the regularity or otherwise of the mother's daily rhythms may affect the developing fetus. If the mother's eating pattern is very irregular—for example, if she snatches a hamburger at an odd time in her working day—then the irregular changes in the amount of glucose crossing to the fetus may be confusing. In the next chapter we will see how maternal nutrition can alter the development and growth of the fetus. Marked malnutrition results in growth retardation. It is also possible that irregular patterns of maternal feeding may affect the development of those parts of the fetal brain that control feeding behavior. We need more research to uncover the links between the mother's behavioral patterns during pregnancy and the development of the fetal brain.

We have seen how fetal behavior was altered by contractures of the uterus. The fetus clearly responds to compression by the uterine muscle and the accompanying changes in the passage of oxygen across the placenta. One night sometime just before delivery in pregnant baboons and monkeys, contractures switch to the strong short-lived contractions of the uterus that are characteristic of the birth process. This switch only lasts a few hours the first time it occurs, and then uterine activity switches back to the contracture type. Each night in the six or seven days immediately before delivery the switch recurs. In monkeys this period of repeated contractions increases each night as delivery approaches. In Chapter 13 we will see that similar patterns of uterine contraction activity almost certainly occur in pregnant women. This pattern of uterine muscle contraction would be able to set the fetal clock to the outside world even before birth.

Several other influences may also help to bring the fetus into synchrony with his mother's day/night patterns before he is born. We have seen that sounds and other sensory information penetrate the uterus. The changes in noise around the mother, her eating habits, her patterns of exercise and relaxation all produce effects that the fetus can monitor. Taken together, this information may enable the fetus to develop his own time-keeping system before he is born, another important preparation for life after birth.

Shift-work may be necessary in some occupations but it does take a toll on the shift-worker. Switching shifts frequently can really confuse the internal clock. It is very likely that the fetus of a pregnant woman shares in the misalignment of internal and external cues if she changes shifts or takes a transatlantic flight. If she gets jet lag, so probably does her baby. The influences of changing environment on development have also been studied in premature newborn babies. When the environment around the baby has carefully controlled rhythmic components such as lighting, touching, and feeding times, the premature baby thrives better and in general is released from the hospital earlier. So, when the baby is in tune with his environment, growth and development are improved.

There are important lessons in all this for the good management of a pregnancy. Regularity of habit—eating, sleeping, work, relaxation—will give the baby a better chance to develop normally. The fetus is a pretty conservative little person who likes things the way he knows them. He doesn't like change, is not fond of surprises, and would in general rather be left to get on with things his own way.

Chapter 10

FETAL GROWTH

Growth is the only evidence of Life.

Cardinal John Henry Newman

Growth of a living organism occurs when there is a net increase in the number of cells and cell constituents. The normal growth of the fetus involves an ordered sequential progress of cell division, cell movement, cell adhesion changes, and cell death. In normal fetal growth and development there is a continuous interaction between the genetic regulators on the chromosomes (the genome) and the environment. The two are often distinguished as nature (genome) and nurture (environment). The potential of the genome is constantly being modified by environmental factors. The genome is responsible for the production of the instructions to cells to produce regulator messenger molecules. These regulators act on cells, usually via receptor molecules, to enable target cells to respond to growth-promoting factors. The signals may be either stimulatory or inhibitory to growth. Growth should be distinguished from differentiation. In general, the processes of growth and differentiation do not take place at the same time, and are incompatible. The cell cycle—manufacture of basic cell constituents, and the duplication of chromosomes—will cease when the cell begins to differentiate to perform its specific tasks.

In the very earliest stages of the life of an embryo, the ordered sequence of growth and differentiation can be adversely affected by toxic compounds in the embryo's environment. These toxic compounds are collectively called teratogens. Teratogens alter the balance of growth and differentiation, and have a very wide range of effects that vary according to the stage of development at which they affect the embryo. The drug thalidomide is a powerful teratogen. It was used extensively by pregnant women in the 1960s to treat the uncomfortable morning sickness of early pregnancy. The results were disastrous. Embryos exposed to thalidomide that had crossed the placenta at critical times in early development suffered abnormal growth of their developing limbs. The extent of the deformity, and whether both the arms and the legs were affected, depended on the precise time of development that the embryo was exposed to the drug. This is another example of the existence of critical and susceptible phases of embryonic development. Most of the deformities were horrifying, condemning otherwise healthy children to lives of extreme frustration and difficulty.

Growth and development represents a precise program of gene activation and suppression occurring in an orderly sequence. The sequence is very important. Omission of crucial steps at a specific time may lead to irreversible damage. Many tissues seem to lose their ability to undergo critical changes after a particular time window has passed. In the human fetus it has been calculated that forty-two cell divisions have to be completed by the time of birth. Tissues appear to count the number of divisions they have completed, so that they know at what stage they are in the overall scheme of the developmental program. This way the correct steps can be taken at the correct time. The orderly sequence of developmental events is fundamental to normal fetal growth. Particular groups of cells appear to play a role in organizing the growth and specialization of major structures. For example, each wing of a chick embryo contains a group of cells called the "progress zone." There is considerable evidence that a developmental clock is located in the embryonic progress zone. If the progress zone of a young undifferentiated limb that is just beginning to form in one chick embryo is transplanted to a wing that is already well formed on another chick embryo, a second wing will be formed at the end of the first already completed wing. In contrast, if the undifferentiated progress zone is replaced by the progress zone of an already formed wing, there is little differentiation. It is as if the progress zone from the wing that has already differentiated has sent its instructions off at the appropriate time and cannot repeat the performance.

While the genome—the genetic regulatory system—of each particular fetus is very important, the environment in which the fetus grows also plays a critical role. Non-genetic constraints imposed by the mother on fetal growth are very important. For example, it has been shown that genetically large fetuses do not grow to their proper size if in an especially small environment.

In the 1930s a very famous and simple study was performed in which large shire horses were bred with Shetland ponies. Although the genetic make-up of the fetuses was similar, the foal born to the shire mother when the father was a Shetland was much larger than the foal born to the Shetland mother when the father was a shire horse. This is not really so surprising. It was assumed that the larger mother with a larger uterus, and presumably a larger blood supply to the placenta, was more likely to permit the fetus to grow to his maximum potential. However, there is a small scientific flaw in this early and very graphic study. The genetic component of the foal will be different if his mother is a shire, a large breed, and the father a Shetland, a small breed, compared with the genetic material the foal would have from the other pairing. For this reason the study has been repeated in pigs. Two strains of pigs were chosen, mini-pigs that weigh about 80 pounds and normal pigs that weigh 400 pounds when fully grown. When embryos in which both parents are normal pigs were transplanted to sows of the miniature pig variety, the piglets born were about half the size of the piglets from similar normal-size embryos transplanted to the normal-size pigs. In this more recent study, genetic material of the embryos was the same in both groups. The factor that differed was the maternal environment.

Maternal nutrition is a major factor affecting fetal growth. The relationship between mother and her developing fetus is partly parasitic. The fetus is a drain on his mother's nutrients. This is not a problem as long as his mother maintains a good, well-balanced diet. However, if his mother is short of nutrients, the fetus begins to compete for materials that are in short supply. Nature has so arranged things that the next generation has a powerful say in how the mother's nutrients are used in times of shortage. The regulatory mechanisms of the mother's tissues ensure that her brain gets all the glucose and other nutrients that it needs. However, next to the mother's brain, the fetus is second in line. There are many maternal and fetal regulatory systems that ensure that, after the maternal brain, the fetus is the last to suffer from any shortages. In famine situations, for instance, the birth weights of babies, although reduced, can be remarkably well-maintained. The German occupation of Holland during World War II caused prolonged famine. Extensive studies on babies born in Holland during that time confirmed the order of partition of maternal nutrients: first the maternal brain and then the fetal requirements.

There are many other environmental factors that will affect fetal growth, including cigarette smoking, living at high altitudes where the amount of oxygen in the air is decreased, chronic and acute maternal infections, drugs (both prescription drugs and drugs-of-abuse), and very high temperatures. Many of these factors exhibit their effects by reducing the blood flow to the uterus, which, if decreased, will also decrease the delivery of nutrients and oxygen going to the fetus and placenta. Eventually this reduction will lead to intrauterine growth retardation.

Fetal growth appears to slow down in the last few weeks of pregnancy. It is unclear why this happens. One suggestion is that the fetus is getting short of nutrients, that he is outgrowing the ability of the placenta to provide, and that there is now a contest between dangerous deprivation in the uterus and delivery. Hippocrates held this view in 600 B.C., but the available scientific data do not support this idea—at least not in a normal pregnancy. There is an abnormality in sheep in which pregnancy may last double the normal length of time, and yet the fetus continues to grow. This observation scarcely supports the view that the placenta cannot support continued growth after the end of normal pregnancy—in the sheep at least. The slowing of the growth rate at the end of pregnancy more likely suggests that the fetal tissues are concentrating their efforts developing their specialized capabilities, preparing for the challenge of adapting to a new world, and are not so interested in merely growing. After all, size is not everything.

When we consider fetal growth we should remember that the fetus is made up of different components; protein, fat, and carbohydrate. A gram of one of these components may not be as useful as a gram of another. Some species such as humans and guinea pigs are born with a very high fat content and others such as sheep and monkeys have very little fat. Fat is the most efficient way to store energy for times of need. Fetuses that have stored up fat during fetal life have been indulging in a type of "lay-away" policy.

There is some suggestion that our fetal dietary history and the amount of fat we put on in childhood will determine how fat we are for the rest of our lives. We do not yet know exactly to what extent these considerations apply to life before birth. If there is a prenatal effect it would be interesting to know how much of the effect is genetic and how much is due to specific features of the environment in the uterus. We need to know whether the mother can eat too much and pass too much glucose and other nutrients to her fetus, thereby affecting his growth patterns into the newborn period. In addition, it is possible that the amount of activity expended in the uterus can affect his weight distribution, as it certainly does after birth. It would be very useful to have some clue as to the factors both prenatal and postnatal, that predispose to obesity, and to know which intrauterine effects persist after birth. There are several reasons for watching weight gain in pregnancy. In addition to potential adverse effects on the fetus, excessive weight gain during pregnancy is correlated with increased maternal blood pressure.

We have seen that the mother does everything to protect the growth of her baby, short of depriving her own central nervous system. In a similar way, the fetus will do everything he can to maintain the growth of his own brain. If the supply of oxygen to the fetus becomes short for any reason, the fetus sets in action regulatory mechanisms that maintain, and even increase, the blood supply to his brain at the expense of other less vital tissues such as his skin. A similar re-distribution of blood flow will take place if the fetus becomes short of nutrients. Everything is done to minimize damage to his brain.

As a result of these compensatory mechanisms, even in pregnancies where growth retardation is pronounced, the head and brain suffer least. This brain-sparing is clearly demonstrated when we compare the circumference of the fetal head to the circumference of the fetal abdomen. In growth retardation, the ratio of head circumference to abdominal circumference is increased. In other words the growth rate of the head and brain is less retarded than the growth of the abdomen. Usually the length of the baby is not much affected by intrauterine growth retardation. These changes in the proportions of the body reflect the compensatory mechanisms the fetus has called into play. In addition, the weight of the placenta is relatively protected.

Throughout pregnancy the nutritional needs of the placenta for normal growth and function have to be taken into account. In all species, the placenta grows faster than the fetus in the early stages of pregnancy. In this way the placenta can develop its ability to provide the fetus with all the nutrients he needs when he begins to grow very fast in the last third of pregnancy. If anything happens to retard the growth of the placenta in the first half of pregnancy the fetus will grow more slowly when the time comes for him to put on his maximum weight, as it is the placenta's job to transport everything necessary for fetal growth from the mother to the fetus. If there is a problem with placental growth, there will be a problem with fetal growth.

In normal pregnancies, there is a correlation at birth between the weight of the placenta and the weight of the baby. However, there is a two-way interaction between the fetus and the placenta that can cause competition in times of shortage of nutrients. The placenta is nearest to the source of maternal nutrients that must cross the placenta to get to the fetus. Thus, there is possibility for competition in situations of shortage.

An interesting recent study of old records from the beginning of this century in England has thrown considerable light on the role of the placenta and on how our intrauterine lives may affect us for the whole of our life after birth. In this study it was shown that several forms of cardiovascular disease in adult life were related to the baby's birth weight. Other factors such as social class, parental income, etc., were ruled out by grouping the individuals studied into similar groups for these factors. Within any one group, the incidence of cardiovascular disease increased in the individuals who were growth-retarded at birth. The correlation of disease in later life and intrauterine growth retardation was further high-lighted by the apparent increase in risk in those babies who were small in relation to the size of their placenta. When the placenta is relatively large for the size of the newborn baby, this is about the strongest indication that the baby was short of nutrients during development and fetal growth suffered more than placental growth. All this underlines how important it is to try to give every child the best start possible by helping him to grow to his full potential in the uterus before birth.

Growth retardation of the type in which the fetus compromises his body to protect his brain is a clear indication that such a growth-retarded fetus was not in the ideal environment throughout pregnancy. It is always necessary to determine if he has succeeded in protecting his brain and vital organs. This type of growth retardation is called asymmetric growth retardation because all tissues are not uniformly affected. The real danger is not so much intrauterine growth retardation but intrauterine brain retardation. How the newborn baby, child, and adult perform in our complex and demanding world will depend on how well his brain has developed. The brain is the secret weapon of the human race. Its proper functioning depends upon the well-being of each member of the species.

If growth is restricted during the early stages of fetal life when the cells are dividing rapidly to form the stem-cells from which the various tissues will be formed, the newborn baby will be uniformly small because all the tissues of his body will weigh less. This type of symmetrical growth retardation is, in many ways, cause for more worry than asymmetric growth retardation, because the number of cells in vital organs like the brain is more likely to have been reduced. Babies who are symmetrically growth-retarded do not have the same capacity to catch up in their weight in the way that asymmetrically growth-retarded babies can.

It is imperative that we find out more about the factors that regulate fetal growth. There is evidence from a study in Sweden that there are second-generation consequences of growth retardation. This Swedish study showed that women who were themselves growth-retarded when they were born had an increased risk of having a growth-retarded baby themselves. Interestingly, they were also at greater risk of having a premature baby. The effect of a mother's birth weight on her baby's birth weight has been confirmed by a study in the United States from the Centers for Disease Control in Atlanta.

We do not yet know the precise long-term effects of intrauterine growth retardation. There may be effects on growth and weight distribution for the rest of an individual's life. One study of the consequences of the Dutch famine suggests that if food deprivation occurs late in pregnancy then the likelihood that the baby will be obese in later life is decreased. By way of complete contrast, if maternal food deprivation occurred in early pregnancy, when the baby reached adult life he was more likely to be obese. Some investigators speculate that this somewhat unexpected finding is explained by a permanent resetting of the centers that regulate appetite in the brains of the fetuses that were nutritionally deprived in early pregnancy. This is an interesting thought, but one that is not yet substantiated by firm data. Such ideas can be likened to islands of supposition joined by bridges of conjecture—more suitable territory for the philosopher than a serious medical scientist.

Chapter 11

BABY ON BOARD—DON'T ABUSE

*Visit the sins of the fathers (and mothers) upon the children unto
the third and fourth generation.*

Book of Common Prayer

An individual might be thought to determine their own lifestyle,
but it is equally true that one's lifestyle determines the nature of the
individual. Our lifestyle is both a consequence of who we are and at
the same time makes us what we are. The widespread occurrence of
heart disease, stomach ulcers, headaches, and other adverse
manifestations of our internal level of stress suggests that many
aspects of our modern lifestyles are not well tuned to our biological
make-up. We are generally not at ease with ourselves. Most of us
do not spend much time planning and working out the shape of the
next nine months. During pregnancy, however, it is very important
that we do precisely that and take a careful look at our lifestyle.
How a pregnant woman eats, how much and how well she sleeps,
how she copes with financial and personal stress over the nine
months of her pregnancy will greatly affect how her baby grows
and develops his skills.

Much of the cause of, and difficulty in dealing with, the
multitude of stressors in modern life lies in the wide diversity of
choices arrayed before us. Our ancestors did not have such a
bewildering array of work and leisure options. Before the advent of
first gas and then electric lighting the choice for the vast majority of

humans was work during the day and rest in the home after dark. You may think that our society has moved on to a higher level of living with freezers, dishwashers, automobiles, even planes to whisk us from Tokyo to Sydney or London to Hong Kong. Yes, our society has moved on but our bodies have not changed at the same rate. Our bodies still work with the same rhythm that was adapted to a fixed and regular lifestyle; sleep, eat, physical work, eat, sleep. In the developed world this rhythm is shattered and held ransom to the fast pace of everyday life. This is equally true for mothers- and fathers-to-be; people who, as we have seen, especially need regularity and calm in their lives.

The multitude of stressful situations that assail us, and the stress responses they generate within the body, are often amplified for the pregnant woman. At some point the mother's stress responses may well begin to directly or indirectly affect her fetus. Even the actions the mother takes to deal with the stress may have effects on the fetus. Thus, smoking to relieve tension, alcohol to provide relaxation, and pharmaceutical agents such as tranquilizers, may all be part of the mother's coping mechanism. It is all too easy for these features of the mother's lifestyle to become harmful to the normal development of the fetus, and all too common for women to ignore these serious dangers.

Our knowledge of the physiology of the body's stress responses has grown considerably in the last few years. Scientists distinguish between the external stressful event and the internal response of the individual to the stressful situation. It is unfortunate that in everyday talk we usually refer to both the external initiating event and the body's response to it with the same word, stress. It is better to distinguish between these related but separate issues. We should call the cause of stress a stressor. The stressors to which we are exposed may be psychological, for example financial worry, or physical, such as a broken bone or a major hemorrhage. The body's response to the stressor is best called the stress response.

When it is the mother who is experiencing stress, the stressor (cause) usually acts on the fetus indirectly, as it results in a stress response. It is the stress response initiated by the mother's body that may adversely affect the fetus. For example, financial worry will not affect the fetus directly (unless it causes an insufficient diet or prenatal care, etc.). However, money worries may lead to an increased secretion of stress-related hormones by the mother. One of these hormones, adrenaline, has very pronounced effects on the mother's cardiovascular system. One action of adrenaline is to decrease blood flow to the uterus and hence to the placenta. In this way the fetus suffers indirectly as a result of his mother's stress responses. If the mother cannot avoid the specific stressor, it is important for her to be provided with the necessary social and psychological support so that she may cope with it as best she can. It is the mother's stress response that is potentially harmful to the fetus. The fetus will get a better chance in life if his mother can have nine months free of money concerns and other major worries.

The stressful situation may also prompt the mother to smoke. The tobacco industry plays on tobacco's ability to soothe frazzled nerves. This may indeed be true but smoking is not a natural way of dealing with stressful situations. One has to learn the habit. If a woman has become dependent on taking a smoke when she is stressed, she is likely to use cigarettes to relieve stressful situations during pregnancy. Cigarette smoking harms the fetus in many ways. Nicotine has been shown to have a powerful constricting action on the maternal uterine arteries. Thus, when a pregnant woman smokes, the blood flow to the placenta declines. As we have already seen, the mother's stress response already may have resulted in hormonally induced reduction of blood flow to the placenta. This unwanted effect of nicotine represents an added assault on the fetus. A double whammy!

Tobacco smoke contains a high concentration of the gases carbon monoxide and carbon dioxide. When the mother inhales these gases with the tobacco smoke the percentage of oxygen in the maternal lungs is decreased. The amount of oxygen in maternal blood falls and hence the amount of oxygen available for transfer to the fetus across the placenta decreases. The oxygen going to the fetus is already lowered because of decreased blood flow to the placenta as a result of stress hormones and nicotine. So now we have a third way in which the fetus' oxygen supply is reduced by smoking. A triple whammy for the fetus.

As if these three reasons for a decreased supply of oxygen that occurs during a smoking bout were not bad enough, the presence of carbon monoxide in the air the mother inhales poses a separate and rather long-term danger. Carbon monoxide is the gas formed when materials are not completely burned. It is present in high concentrations in tobacco smoke. The ancient Greeks and Romans actually used carbon monoxide as a means of criminal execution. Carbon monoxide combines with hemoglobin to form a compound that cannot transport oxygen. Once formed in the red cells, this compound is only very slowly broken down. Following a smoking bout it hangs around for a long time. In this way smoking will reduce the capacity of red blood cells to carry oxygen around the mother and her fetus. This effect of carbon monoxide can also occur as a result of passive smoking if the people around the pregnant mother are filling the air with carbon monoxide. Carbon monoxide also comprises six percent or more of the exhaust emissions of automobiles. At low speeds automobiles produce large amounts of toxic exhaust fumes, so the danger is even greater in exhaust-fume-laden cities such as London, Los Angeles, and Tokyo where traffic speeds may be down as low as five miles an hour.

If at the same time as the mother smokes and her secretion of stress hormones is increased, the financial worry leads to an excessive consumption of alcohol, then the alcohol in the mother's blood may cause even further decreases in blood flow to the uterus. In addition, alcohol will cross the placenta and enter the fetus' blood. If the concentration built up in the fetus exceeds certain limits, damage to the growing and dividing fetal cells will occur. The most sensitive cells in the developing fetus are nerve cells. Once damaged, nerve cells cannot be replaced. Major nervous system deformities have been reported following alcoholic binges early in pregnancy. It is now clear that the high concentrations of alcohol in the fetus' blood during the critical periods of organ development may result in a fundamental abnormality of the nervous system, for which the developing fetus never compensates.

Alcohol's effects on fetuses in late pregnancy have been studied extensively, particularly by the late Dr. John Patrick from London, Ontario. Dr. Patrick showed that alcohol will inhibit breathing movements by the fetus. It appears that alcohol in the fetal blood gets to the fetal brain and stimulates the excessive production of prostaglandins by the cells that regulate fetal breathing. This observation is important for at least two reasons. First, it shows how susceptible fetal brain cells are to alcohol. Second, as we have seen, fetal breathing movements are critical to the normal development of the lungs of the fetus. So it seems that fetuses repeatedly exposed to high levels of alcohol may have impaired lung, as well as brain, development. The lung impairment may not be life-threatening but will certainly result in the baby not reaching his full potential as a child and adult.

The repeated exposure of the developing fetal brain to alcohol is one of the most extensively investigated examples of the effects of substance abuse during pregnancy. In 1982 one study reported that the incidence of heavy drinking by mothers was around nine percent of pregnant women in the United States. Repeated exposure of the fetus to alcohol can lead to the Fetal Alcohol Syndrome, first described in 1973. The face of the affected baby has a characteristic appearance: the eyes are narrowed, the bridge of the nose is flattened, and the nose is short. The upper lip is thin, the ears are set low and not exactly opposite each other. Alcohol is a toxic compound. If the dividing cells of the early embryo are exposed to high concentrations of alcohol at critical times of their development, damage may occur to the heart, kidneys, and nerves and muscles as well as the brain. After the early phase of cell differentiation is completed, alcohol is still harmful to the fetus as the delayed division of cells causes stunted growth. Mothers who drink a lot of alcohol tend to eat less and, therefore, the fetus can be deprived of major nutrients, adding to the impairment of growth.

Children who were exposed to excessive amounts of alcohol when in the uterus often have a decreased attention span, are likely to be hyperactive, and are more easily distracted. They lack the integrating functions of their brain that allow them to understand cause and effect. Many children exposed to excessive alcohol while in the uterus fall foul of the law because they steal and lie, often quite openly. They do not attempt to hide their crimes, as they do not fully understand the nature or consequences of their actions. The possible long-term behavioral effects of alcohol recently received much attention in the days before the execution of Robert Alton Harris in the California gas chamber. Harris' mother drank heavily during Robert Harris' life before birth. His defense lawyers claimed that the effects of the alcohol had left him unable to understand the consequences of his actions. It is beyond the scope of this book to consider the legal, moral, and ethical issues of the legal plea of diminished responsibility. However, what is clear is that society does pay for its inattention to the long-term consequences of an adverse intrauterine environment. The cost of research into the causal mechanisms of abnormal prenatal influences of alcohol, cocaine, tobacco, and other noxious agents will ultimately be repaid to society in several ways. It is to be hoped that a better understanding of the consequences of these lifestyles will help mothers to avoid them. If not, the pharmaceutical industry may be able to fashion drug therapies for use at periods of critical susceptibility. Certainly, the cost of treatment centers is far in excess of the amounts of money currently being spent on research into prevention of alcohol and drug abuse.

In recent years we have learned a great deal about the ways alcohol affects the developing fetal brain. We have seen that the fetus shows clearly defined patterns of sleep and wakefulness, with periods of REM sleep-type activity. These patterns are gradually maturing as the fetal brain matures. The brain waves of the fetus exposed to alcohol are different in their patterns from the normal fetus. The amount of time the fetus spends breathing or in REM sleep decreases. As we have seen, the amount of fetal breathing is critical for normal lung development, and the patterning of REM sleep is both an index as well as a regulator of normal fetal brain development.

Alcohol crosses the placenta very rapidly so that the concentrations in the blood of the fetus and mother very quickly become equal during a drinking bout. Both the fetus and the placenta are deficient in the enzymes that metabolize and remove alcohol from the blood. Thus, alcohol that gets across the placenta to the fetus is present in the fetus for a long time. This is one example of a situation in which the placenta does not protect the fetus. The fetus has an added complication in his attempt to get rid of the alcohol that he has unwillingly consumed as a result of his mother's drinking. In addition to passing through the placenta, alcohol passes from mother to fetus across the fetal membranes into the amniotic fluid. Also, alcohol that has passed across the placenta into the fetal blood is excreted in the fetal urine and out into the amniotic fluid. Alcohol that has contaminated the amniotic fluid by these routes has no rapid means of escape and remains there and may slowly return again into the fetal blood to provide another exposure. One of the major harmful products of alcohol is acetaldehyde derived from alcohol by enzyme action; luckily for the fetus, his liver and placenta are not very good at converting alcohol to acetaldehyde. Therefore, the fetus is to some extent protected. These intriguing differences between the metabolism of the fetus and his mother merit further exploration if we are to understand Fetal Alcohol Syndrome. Again, it shows that we must study the fetus to see how the fetus works; we can't guess correctly all the time by knowing how the adult body deals with a problem.

Adults who drink alcohol in large amounts at regular intervals become tolerant of some of its intoxicating effects; their brains do not show the same effects of alcohol consumption as the brains of those who do not drink alcohol regularly. It seems as if the fetus also can develop a tolerance. In one study, the fetus of a mother who drank heavily and regularly was observed. The mother's alcohol concentrations were about five times the legal limit for driving, and yet the fetal breathing rhythms were normal. Features such as memory and judgement are impaired in chronic alcoholics who show tolerance to alcohol. They have paid a great price for their ability to tolerate alcohol without appearing to get drunk. We do not yet know the significance of this, and what long-term price these babies of heavy alcohol consumers may be forced to pay.

Coping with stressors in our lives may tempt a rush to the pharmacist. Over-the-counter drugs are a convenience that does not require the expense of a consultation with the physician. The body metabolizes drugs differently during pregnancy; drugs can cross the placenta and harm the fetus. Yet, pregnant women often do not even tell the pharmacist that they are pregnant. Tranquilizers and other agents that enhance the ability to cope have features in common with all drugs developed for clinical use.

Drugs used in the treatment of disease are simply chemical compounds that interact with the normal cell processes that occur all the time. They owe their effectiveness to their similarity to natural compounds that we produce in our own bodies. The value of each drug is directly related to the power with which it increases or decreases the specific cellular processes involved in the disease in question. Some compounds used in the treatment of diseases are the actual molecule produced in the body. Thus if you have a very bad reaction to a bee sting, so that your breathing airways are constricted and you cannot breathe, your physician may give you an injection of adrenaline, which naturally occurs in the body. Adrenaline will attach to receptors on the muscles surrounding your airways and stop them from contracting. As a direct result, your airways will dilate and enable you to breathe more freely.

Alternatively, the pharmaceutical chemist may alter the shape of the adrenaline molecule a little to produce a similar but more powerful compound, a designer drug. One major difference between normal transmitters (naturally occurring drugs) and designer drugs is that the effect of designer drugs may be much more prolonged than the effect of the body's naturally secreted transmitters. Specially synthesized drugs may also have a greater effect on the body than the natural transmitters because the designer drug may have a greater capability to attach to the receptor on the target cell than the body's own molecule. Designer drugs may also have wider effects than the related naturally occurring compounds because the synthetic molecules may bind to a wider range of receptors, thus giving rise to side effects. Some drugs alter the balance of opposing mechanisms within the body. By so doing, they may be safe at one level and have harmful effects at others.

A good example of all this is the very common drug aspirin, currently being studied in clinical trials to assess its ability to prevent the onset of high blood pressure in pregnancy. The extent of constriction of the blood vessels is the major factor that regulates the blood pressure in both the mother and fetus. As a result of extensive research studies with animals, cells studied in a dish, and with clinical patients, we now know that prostaglandins play an important role in regulating the degree of constriction of blood vessels in many parts of the body including the uterus. We also know that the balance of different prostaglandins shifts from time to time. Thromboxane is a member of the prostaglandin family that is released from the platelets in the blood and stimulates contraction of the small blood vessels. Opposing this constrictor action is prostacyclin, produced by the cells that line the blood vessels. Aspirin promotes the production of prostacyclin over the production of thromboxane. At low levels of aspirin treatment, the effect appears to be very beneficial and can lower maternal blood pressure. If, however, too much aspirin is consumed, unwanted effects such as widespread maternal bleeding may occur, with harmful effects for the fetus. It is unwise for the pregnant mother to consume any drug, unless it is under the supervision and guidance of her physician.

It is the hit-or-miss element in non-prescription drugs that makes them especially dangerous during pregnancy. During pregnancy, the effect of the drug may go on longer than in the non-pregnant woman. Thus, the fetus may be exposed to the direct and indirect effects of the drug for a long time, and there may be undesirable side effects. Also, without the advice of a professional who knows about how drugs interact during pregnancy, the drug may be administered in inappropriate doses, or inappropriately combined with other drugs. Once again: "If in doubt, leave it out." Or, as Voltaire said, "Abstain."

Every concern regarding the effects on the fetus of prescription drugs taken in pregnancy can be magnified ten-fold when we consider street drugs. Drugs-of-abuse are bad news because they have powerful effects on important cell functions. In particular they alter important functions in brain cells. It is this very property—the ability to alter the function of the brain—that makes the drug addict want the drug. How much more, then, are drugs-of-abuse bad news for the fetus!

The "crack" cocaine explosion has had tragic consequences for a whole generation of unborn children. Cocaine is a powerful drug that enhances the effects of the group of transmitters known as catecholamines. These transmitters play a critical role in the stress response to danger. Cocaine produces its effects by stopping the removal of the catecholamine transmitters from the nerve terminals where they are secreted, thereby increasing and prolonging their effects. Several studies have shown that the concentration of noradrenaline (one of the catecholamine family) is increased in the blood of the babies of cocaine-abusing mothers. These increased levels of cocaine and catecholamines in the blood and brain affect the heart, causing it to beat faster, irritate the central nervous system, and produce immediate and long-term harmful effects. Catecholamines, generally, are removed quickly from the sites at which they are produced. Following a dose of cocaine, the catecholamines act for much longer on maternal and fetal blood vessels, and nerve cells. Cocaine may increase the level of excitement but it does so at a cost both to the mother who willingly took the cocaine and the fetus who unwillingly suffered the consequences.

Cocaine constricts the uterine arteries. As a result the fetus becomes short of oxygen. Even with relatively modest doses of cocaine the fetus becomes severely hypoxic (short of oxygen). The episode of hypoxemia may last for several minutes. Because this action is in the mother it is not even necessary for the drug to get to the fetus to have this harmful affect. Cocaine does, however, cross the placenta readily and will have direct effects on the fetus as well. One of the striking effects that cocaine has is to cause an increase in fetal limb movements. It is particularly dangerous for the fetus to move around too much when he is short of oxygen. As we have seen, even when moderately short of oxygen, the normal fetus suspends breathing and limb movements as a conservation maneuver. When cocaine acts on the fetal brain to stimulate movement in times of oxygen deprivation, the fetus will generate significant amounts of lactic acid as a result of the muscle contraction, and the acidity in the fetal blood increases. If the bouts of hypoxia and acidity are repeated, as they often are in addicts with repeated doses over short periods of time, there may be permanent damage to the fetal brain.

The cocaine that has crossed the placenta acts on the fetal brain to wake up the fetus, so the overall effect of repeated doses of cocaine is to disturb the sleep/wakefulness patterns that would normally occur. Consequently, it is not surprising that the newborn baby exposed repeatedly to cocaine before birth is highly irritable and difficult to quiet down. He is often in almost continuous motion. His brain has become totally confused. His limb muscles are tightly contracted for long periods of time. As if these observations were not disturbing enough, we do not yet know the long-term effects of maternal cocaine abuse on the structure of the brains of these unfortunate babies.

Cocaine disturbs the normal patterns of fetal breathing. It is to be expected that the problems associated with abnormal development of the centers in the brain that regulate breathing in the fetus and newborn place cocaine-exposed babies at a high risk for SIDS.

Another issue regarding cocaine is worth mentioning. Dr. James Woods in Rochester, New York has shown that cocaine has much more marked effects on the adult cardiovascular system in the pregnant state than in the non-pregnant state. This enhanced responsiveness to cocaine appears to be caused by the high concentrations of progesterone that are produced during pregnancy. These observations show how important it is to study both the fetus and pregnant mother. We cannot extrapolate information obtained in non-pregnant subjects and assume that the fetus or his mother will respond in the same way.

Many forms of substance abuse are associated with intrauterine growth retardation. Intrauterine brain retardation also occurs because heroin, morphine, and cocaine abuse by pregnant women have been shown to lead to smaller head circumference of the baby, presumably due to the smaller brain. This decreased head circumference is still present at two years of age. We must remain concerned that critical phases of brain development may have been missed or have occurred out of sequence. The normal sequence of events is a major factor that shapes the child's future abilities.

Before we leave the issue of maternal lifestyle it is important to assess the effects of maternal work, sleep, and exercise on the development of the fetus. Nothing currently available from a physician improves uterine blood flow better than real rest. Rest is extremely important especially when twins are present, as the demands on the mother are doubled—as they may be after birth.

Pregnancy need not interrupt a normal exercise routine. In developing societies women frequently continue heavy physical work right through pregnancy. However, high-intensity exercise does direct blood away from the uterus to the working muscles. Therefore, prolonged high-intensity exercise can leave the placenta deprived of oxygen and nutrients contained in the blood. In someone used to a particular level of exercise, the body is well able to cope at that level during pregnancy. General activity as well as prenatal exercises to strengthen the muscles of the pelvis and prepare for the process of birth are important.

The American College of Obstetricians has guidelines for the maximum intensity that a pregnant woman should exercise. The level of exercise should not exceed the target rate set for each individual according to their weight, age, and exercise capacity when non-pregnant. Safe levels are best worked out with your obstetrician. Above levels of moderate exercise, changes in fetal heart rate suggest that the fetus is being adversely affected by the exercise. Walking, swimming, and biking are the best aerobic forms of exercise during pregnancy with swimming probably the best. Swimming puts the least strain on the pregnant woman's body.

Dr. James Clapp III, an authority on exercise in pregnancy, believes that the guidelines should be different for women who have exercised regularly before pregnancy and those who have not. He has demonstrated in extensive studies that the body can cope with normal activities during pregnancy. The level of exercise taken when not pregnant need not be changed during pregnancy. However, if very little exercise was done before pregnancy, then the mother-to-be should not attempt vigorous exercise. It is probably wise not to start a particular exercise regimen once pregnancy has started: better to stick to gentle regular walks or swimming.

Thus, we see that our lifestyles are indeed just that, styles for life. If we also pay attention to the general health and social balance of our children we will not only be doing the best for them, but in turn they are likely to become considerate parents and pass on their advantages to the next generation. "Couch potatoes," for instance, are not good role models for their children. Parents who indulge in too much alcohol, smoke, or take recreational drugs may affect the lives of their children as well as their grandchildren.

Chapter 12

A Time To Be Born

To every thing there is a season, and a time to every purpose under heaven: A time to be born, and a time to die.

Ecclesiastes, Chapter 3, v. 1

The normal birth of a healthy baby that has gone full term and is properly matured is the single most important factor that determines whether the baby will get off to a good start and adapt well to his new environment outside the uterus. How the birth process is controlled, who decides the time to be born, and how long pregnancy will last are questions that have long puzzled scientists. Some answers are now being offered by various research groups around the world. The more we learn about the birth process, the better all involved are able to prepare for and enjoy it. It helps enormously when the parents, the family, and the medical caregivers have a unified approach to an event that is the most natural of processes. A normal birth is a joyful and uniting experience for a whole family. Problems at birth on the other hand can lead to all kinds of tensions, and a baby can be propelled into a world full of anxiety. So, for the sake of both the baby and the family, it is essential to do everything we can to make birth as uncomplicated as possible.

It is most helpful if everyone involved has a shared understanding of how the fetus and mother are functioning in late pregnancy. In the last twenty years, researchers have provided us with some remarkable and intimate insights into the nature of the birth process. We have come to better understand what is happening in this partnership between mother and fetus. The birth process is an act of teamwork. Under normal circumstances, four or five weeks before he is born the baby takes control of the process. The fetus has his own program that tells him how long pregnancy should last. When this program is activated he passes the information on to his mother. He calls upon several systems in his mother to help him successfully complete the birth process, but the initial timing is his. Having played such an important role in the timing of our entry into this world it is a pity that we do not remember more about it. Fortunately research can now give us some firm insights into the whole process.

Nature has developed a precise program that controls a baby's development in the uterus. As we have seen, in the forty weeks of pregnancy many vital systems must mature to an independent state. As if developing independent capabilities were not complex enough, during this time the fetus must take care of all the problems that are peculiar to his existence in the uterus at the same time. We have discussed several of these critical needs of the fetus, for example, how the fetus alters the blood flow to different regions of his body if he gets short of oxygen and how he normally makes breathing movements in a periodic manner rather than continuously. Limbs, organs, nervous system, heart and blood system, endocrine control systems: all these have to be matured to the correct level before a successful transition to an independent life outside the uterus can be guaranteed. Delayed or incorrect development of any of these vital fetal systems may result in great risks for the baby. Being born prematurely, before all the normal preparations have been completed, can also create problems for him.

The maintenance of a normal pregnancy for around nine months is a wonderful and awesome biological process. The fetus is tolerated by the mother as he grows and matures according to a precisely scheduled program. Several considerations suggest that the mother's body would normally want to reject this foreign invader. He removes nutrients and oxygen from her blood. At times he moves around incessantly, making her quite uncomfortable. He grows so that the uterus is stretched to several times its non-pregnant size. Fortunately, powerful mechanisms exist to maintain the pregnancy even in the presence of these marked changes in the mother's body. These mechanisms include the hormone progesterone, whose action quiets the spontaneous contractile activity of the uterine muscle. Pregnancy allows time for the baby to grow and mature, and for the mother to adjust her physiology to this new person who will shortly delight the family. Before the newborn baby can join the family, the factors that have maintained the pregnancy for nine long months must be overcome. Deciding that pregnancy has lasted long enough, and that the baby is adequately mature to survive in the outside world, is obviously a critical decision. The tantalizing question has always been whether this decision is made by the mother or the fetus.

Correct timing of birth is necessary because the process of passing from the uterus to the outside world is far from being straightforward. The fetus has to make enormously complicated adjustments to his life-support systems in a very short space of time, during which he becomes a newborn baby. Delays are not possible. Up to the moment of birth the fetus has received all his oxygen from his mother across the placenta. His lungs have been unused and unexpanded. We have seen that he practices using his lungs, but he still has to adjust to filling his lungs with air and oxygen.

At the moment of birth the newborn baby has to stop practicing and begin the real thing. This means reversing many of the rules under which he operated throughout his life as a fetus. No longer can he reckon that if he does nothing at all the oxygen supply from his mother will continue to nourish him adequately under widely differing conditions of oxygen supply. Suddenly he has to work the bellows of his chest, pumping his chest muscles and diaphragm for his very life if his oxygen supply is short. Now, as a newborn baby he must use his lungs to survive. He is born into a lifetime's labor of breathing to stay alive.

In the uterus the fetus has given top priority to his brain right up until the time of birth. He has pumped his most richly oxygenated blood to his brain. He has made sure that his brain has obtained materials for growth even, if necessary, at the expense of other tissues. From the moment of birth he has, as it were, to re-wire the circuit and stop favoring the brain. From now on all the parts of the body (except the lungs) will get blood that is equally oxygenated.

The newborn baby can perform a wide range of clever tricks that endear him to his parents and others around him. He can wave, scream, kick, suck, see, blow bubbles, and much more. These miracles of muscular movement are coordinated in a characteristic baby fashion. At the snip of an umbilical cord, all these new responses to the challenges of his environment have to come into action. So obviously it is vital that the fetus choose the correct time to be born: a time when all his vital systems are mature enough to survive in his new environment, when all his systems are set at "Go."

A major breakthrough in this direction is the discovery that it is the fetus who decides the time to be born. How this discovery was made is in itself an intriguing story.

The Greek philosopher, physician, and scientist Hippocrates, who lived in the seventh century B.C., firmly believed that the baby decides when the birth process will begin. He said, "When the child has grown big and the mother can no longer support him with food, he struggles and breaks forth into the world, free from all bonds." Hippocrates held strongly to the view that the signal that begins the process is a failure of the placenta to keep up with the increasing nutritional needs of the fetus. In the 1930s Sir Joseph Barcroft, Professor and Chairperson of Physiology at Cambridge University in England, was the first to attempt to use direct experiments with pregnant sheep to assess various functions of the fetus, while the fetal lamb was still in the uterus. Sir Joseph developed techniques for placing small catheters in blood vessels in the fetal lamb and the pregnant ewe under anesthesia. With these catheters in place, Sir Joseph could take samples simultaneously from both the maternal and fetal blood and measure the amounts of oxygen and other molecules that these samples contained.

As a result of his studies Sir Joseph proposed that as the fetus grows, his needs for oxygen gradually exceed the ability of his mother to provide enough oxygen through the placenta. Sir Joseph viewed the normal birth process as a race between, on the one hand, the danger of the fetus dying while still in the uterus due to lack of oxygen, and on the other hand being born before the oxygen supply gave up. Barcroft wrote many scientific papers about the environment in which the fetus lives and develops. He was particularly interested in the fetal brain and would have supported more recent findings that the fetal brain is active and capable while still in the uterus. The naming of the 1990s as the "Decade of the Brain" would have appealed to Joseph Barcroft. However, such has been the speed of progress that even he would be amazed by the observations that researchers have been able to make over the last twenty years using modern high-technology instrumentation and sensors in experimental animals and pregnant women. He would have marvelled to find out just how active and in control of its own destiny the fetal brain has been shown to be.

The ideas of Hippocrates two millennia ago and those of Barcroft fifty years ago, were similar in suggesting that the fetal awareness of failing supplies of life-supporting substances produced the need to be born. Hippocrates believed that the fetus can sense when his nutrient supply is getting low. Barcroft considered that the critical condition that the fetus monitors is lack of oxygen. These views introduce the concept of the fetal brain as a decision-making computer, analyzing input and acting accordingly. However, the ideas put forward by both Hippocrates and Barcroft had three major deficiencies. First, neither of them had conclusive experimental evidence to prove that the fetus runs short of oxygen, nutrients, or any other factor, at the end of pregnancy. Hippocrates did no experimental studies and Barcroft lacked the ability we now possess to study pregnant animals over several days in order to observe significant trends as pregnancy progresses. Second, neither of them put forward any ideas on the precise mechanism the fetus might use to sense impending danger. Finally, even if the fetus can sense that he is getting short of vital materials, neither of them could describe the specific nature of the mechanisms that the fetus might use to bring about his own birth. Their writings make no mention of the location of the clock, or clocks, that decide that pregnancy has gone on long enough and determine the time to be born.

Because neither Hippocrates nor Barcroft put forward any scientific evidence, their views can only be regarded as guesses at worst, and at best useful hypotheses on which to design experimental studies. It needed years of painstaking research to begin to identify the precise clock mechanism in the fetal brain and locate the process by which the fetus starts things happening. However, the idea of the fetal brain as a decision-making computer was a logical and useful starting point.

In order to understand how the baby decides when to be born, we need information on the nature of the input to the central regulator or computer, and the processes that actually bring about the delivery of the baby, the mechanisms, tools if you like, that the fetus uses. We still know very little about the information the fetus needs to assess before he says to himself "Now's the time to get going!" However, in the last twenty years much has been learned about the central computer and the signals from the fetal brain that start off the birth process.

It took the observation of unusual disease conditions in pregnant women and in pregnant animals to point researchers in the right direction to solve the mystery of the fetal role in the initiation of birth. In 1933 Percy Malpas, an obstetrician, wrote a medical-scientific paper describing the prolongation of human pregnancy that occurs when a fetus is born with part of the brain missing or deformed (anencephaly). In the anencephalic fetus the front portions of the brain have failed to develop and the baby is generally born dead. If the anencephalic baby survives birth he can live only a few hours without the support he derived from his mother through the placenta. Unless other complications are present anencephalic babies are generally born well past the normal expected time of birth. Some researchers took this as the first clue that the critical signals that start the process of birth might have been missing because they were lodged in the part of the fetal brain that was itself missing in the anencephalic baby.

The next clue was provided by veterinarians. In the early 1960s reports began to circulate in the western states of the United States regarding three related naturally occurring situations, two in cows and one in sheep, in each of which the duration of pregnancy was altered. In each case there were similar abnormalities in the fetal brain and fetal endocrine system. In both adult animals and humans, the endocrine system to a very large extent is controlled by the brain. The main pathway of control is through the part of the brain known as the hypothalamus, which lies at the base of the brain and is connected by a special set of blood vessels, the pituitary portal system, to the pituitary gland. The pituitary portal blood system is a private communication pathway between the hypothalamus and the pituitary.

The pituitary controls several other endocrine glands by secreting hormones directly into the blood. The pituitary is the master endocrine gland and controls so many other endocrine glands that it has been called "the conductor of the endocrine orchestra." In the role of conductor, the pituitary tells the other endocrine glands what tune to play, when to play it, how loud or soft, and for how long. Hormonal messengers secreted into the blood by the pituitary pass round the body until they reach their target glands, which have cell surface receptors tuned to receive the specific pituitary hormone. One such system, the one we need to consider in relation to the timing of birth, involves a hierarchy of endocrine glands. The hypothalamus regulates the pituitary by secreting a hormone, corticotropin-releasing hormone (CRH). CRH stimulates the pituitary to secrete adrenocorticotropin (ACTH). ACTH is a hormone that regulates how much of another hormone, cortisol, is secreted by the adrenal cortex. Cortisol from the adrenal regulates the function of several different tissues. Any of these steps can provide opportunities for control of the whole system taken together. They are also a potential cascade that permits rapid and pronounced amplification of the system.

In California near the town of Stockton, a farmer reported that in one herd of Guernsey cows, some cows repeatedly delivered their calves late. Prolonged pregnancy also occurred among a nearby herd of Holstein-Friesian cattle. The veterinary pathologists at the University of California at Davis were able to show that in the affected newborn calves of both of these herds the endocrine hierarchy just described was functioning at a very low level.

At about the same time a very dramatic clue came from the alpine meadows of Idaho. Pregnant sheep, who had eaten a particular plant similar to the skunk cabbage early in their pregnancy, were carrying their lambs well past two hundred days of pregnancy. This degree of prolongation of pregnancy was remarkable because sheep normally give birth at about one hundred fifty days of pregnancy. The fetal lambs of ewes who had eaten the skunk cabbage were not born. They had to be removed surgically from the ewes by cesarean section. Some of these fetal lambs had not been born even as late as two hundred fifty days of pregnancy. A pregnancy lasting two hundred fifty days in sheep is equivalent to a human pregnancy lasting fifteen months instead of the normal nine months. The lamb fetuses that had not delivered had hideous deformities, including just one eye, reminiscent of the mythical character Cyclops. The lamb fetuses also had brain deformities involving the hypothalamus and pituitary. Detailed chemical analysis proved that these deformities were caused by a specific toxic compound in the so-called skunk cabbage. If the embryo was at a critical point of its development when the plant was eaten, the fetal brain developed abnormally. Studies proved that the toxic compound has to reach the fetal brain on the fourteenth day of pregnancy.

All these observations of prolonged pregnancy have one underlying theme. They all suggest involvement of the fetal hypothalamus, pituitary, and adrenal gland in the process of birth. What the signal is, where in the fetus it originates, and when it is given remained questions to be tackled. The time was now right for some controlled experimental animal studies to determine the nature of the abnormality that was causing pregnancy to continue far longer than normal in these situations, namely: human anencephaly, the pituitary and adrenal abnormalities of cattle, and the deformities produced following the consumption of the skunk cabbage by pregnant ewes. Researchers reasoned that if more could be learned about how normal birth starts, we would be in a better position to understand the causes of premature and abnormal birth. Once we know the causes of premature birth, obstetricians will be better placed to prevent premature birth. The high mortality rate might then be decreased, as well as the incidence of long-term damage that many babies experience as a result of being born too soon and too small.

Controlled experimental studies of the fetal brain were begun in the late 1960s. Generally, a medical condition has one primary cause, but in a sick individual the picture is quickly obscured by secondary consequences. Once the secondary processes start, it becomes difficult to decide what is cause and what is effect. To understand the signals that end pregnancy and lead to birth we have to isolate the primary causes from the secondary consequences by careful control of our experiments. If the experiment is to be successful the investigator must try to alter only one factor at a time. The effect of that key central factor, or factors, can then be precisely defined. Experiments had to be designed to test whether it is the fetus or the mother who controls the duration of pregnancy. If, as looked likely, it is the fetus who initiates the birth process then we must try to find the source of the control signal. It would be necessary to test the individual roles of the fetal brain, hypothalamus, pituitary, and adrenals in determining the duration of pregnancy.

These clues strongly suggested, but did not prove, that the fetal pituitary is involved in determining how long pregnancy will last. A series of classical studies was performed by Professor Mont Liggins, an obstetrician from New Zealand while on sabbatic leave at the University of California, Davis. He reasoned that if he could surgically take away the fetal pituitary early in pregnancy he could mimic the prolonged pregnancy that occurs in the much more complex situation of the anencephalic human fetus, the abnormal calves, and the cyclopian fetal lambs. He conducted a series of elegant and precise studies.

Liggins found that when he removed the pituitary gland from fetal sheep at around one hundred fifteen days of pregnancy, pregnancy went on well past its normal length of one hundred fifty days. In separate studies he found that removal of both of the fetal adrenal glands also led to prolongation of pregnancy. So he now had clear experimental evidence that what he needed to focus on was the regulation of the fetal adrenal gland by the hormone

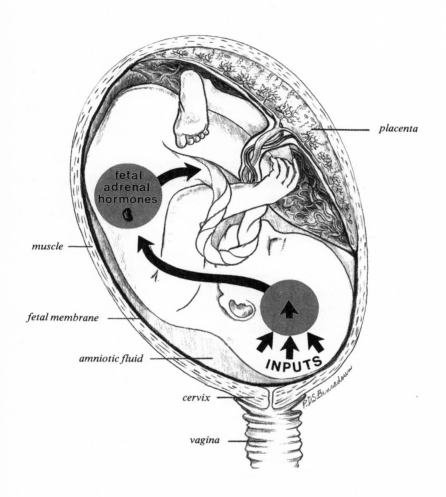

FIGURE 12.1

Control of the birth process by the fetal brain. The brain, the central computer, receives input information and as a result of analysis of this information the brain sends commands to the fetal, placental, and maternal tissues that eventually cause the uterine muscle to contract in the pattern that leads to birth.

adrenocorticotropin (ACTH) secreted by the fetal pituitary. He reasoned that if he reversed the process and stimulated premature growth of the adrenal of the fetal lamb while it was still in the uterus, the duration of the pregnancy would be shortened. So at one hundred twenty days of pregnancy he infused a fetal lamb that was still in the uterus with ACTH to cause the fetal adrenal glands to grow prematurely. The lamb was born within four days. If he missed out a step in the cascade process and infused fetal lambs with cortisol, which is the major product of the adrenal gland, the lambs were born in three days. Fetal lambs infused with saline which he used as a control experiment, did not deliver early; they remained in the uterus and were born at the correct time, around one hundred fifty days of pregnancy. These elegant studies firmly established that in the sheep the fetus is the originator of the signal to be born. The studies also clearly established the fetal pituitary and adrenal system as the major pathway for the signals that initiate the birth process. Professor Liggins' enormous contribution to the body of knowledge of physiology was recognized when Queen Elizabeth II bestowed a knighthood on him in 1991.

The production of ACTH in the fetal lamb is controlled by CRH from the fetal hypothalamus. This hormone is secreted by two paraventricular nuclei, small collections of nerve cells each about the size of a ball-bearing, one on either side of the fetal hypothalamus. Recent studies by Dr. Thomas McDonald and myself at the College of Veterinary Medicine at Cornell University have concentrated on these nuclei. We have shown that if radio frequency waves are used to destroy both of these nuclei in the fetal hypothalamus at 120 days of pregnancy, the pregnancy is prolonged. Working independently, Dr. Peter Gluckman and his team in Auckland, New Zealand have confirmed these findings. Thus the field has been narrowed so that we can pinpoint the paraventricular nuclei as playing a central role in initiating the birth process. This, at last, is clear scientific evidence that the fetal brain plays a key role, probably a decisive role, in determining the length of pregnancy.

There is now a firm body of experimental evidence to show that late in pregnancy, about twenty days before birth, the fetal lamb

begins to increase the secretion of ACTH from his pituitary gland,
stimulating the fetal adrenal cortex to grow and to secrete more
cortisol. ACTH is secreted by the mother's pituitary gland too,
especially at times of stress. Could stress in the mother cause
enough ACTH to be released to influence the fetal adrenal? More
studies concluded that the answer is "No." Maternal ACTH cannot
affect the fetal lamb. ACTH in the blood of the pregnant ewe does
not cross the placenta. Consequently, the fetal adrenal gland is
protected from the effects of changes in maternal ACTH that may
occur as a result of maternal stress. This does not mean that
adverse situations in the mother cannot contribute to premature
birth. As we shall see, there are many ways that an abnormality in
the physiology of the mother can have adverse effects on the baby.
There is much a pregnant mother can do, particularly relating to
lifestyle, to help her baby grow normally and offset the possibility
of premature birth. Later, we will see the ways in which maternal
problems may adversely alter development of the fetus and
increase the risk of premature birth.

Taken together, the series of studies in pregnant sheep show that
as a result of increased activity of the fetal brain, the fetus secretes
more ACTH and cortisol, producing the changes that lead to birth.
The muscle layers of the uterus (the myometrium), are regulated by
both inhibitory and stimulatory regulatory molecules. During
pregnancy the balance is in favor of inhibition of uterine contraction so that the pregnancy will be maintained. At the end of
pregnancy, so that birth may occur, the balance has to be switched
to stimulation. In sheep and other species, the hormone progesterone has an inhibitory effect on the myometrium. In contrast,
estrogens are stimulatory to the myometrium. As the blood from
the fetal lamb passes through the placenta, cortisol in the fetal
blood stimulates the placenta to produce enzymes that convert
progesterone molecules into estrogens. This fall in progesterone
level and associated rise in estrogen production is the first step in
an exquisitely beautiful and precisely timed cascade of effects. The
interactions of the individual components of the cascade show all
the precision and orderliness of a Mozart symphony. As progesterone production by the placenta falls and estrogen production

rises, the balance that has kept the uterine muscle relatively quiet throughout pregnancy begins to change in favor of the stimulatory group of steroids, the estrogens. The signal that started in the fetal brain has been converted to changes in the mother that will stimulate the uterus to contract.

The natural reaction of the mother's body to the presence within her uterus of foreign tissues would be to reject them. We are only now coming to understand just how foreign a body the fetus is, with his totally individual genetic identity from the minute of conception. Much of the energy and skill of maternal function goes to counteract the tendency to reject the growing fetal tissues. As the fetus grows and moves and as the bulge gets bigger and she feels more cumbersome, the mother has to calm the muscle in the uterine wall. The uterine muscle, the myometrium, would naturally tend to contract and expel the little invader. The principal calming agent is the hormone progesterone, which is produced in sufficient quantities to keep the uterus in a state of equilibrium.

The progress of the birth process is initially very gradual. Many physical preparations must be made before the final onset of well-established labor. At the beginning, several processes that stimulate the uterine muscle to contract, such as the production of prostaglandin, are brought into effect. Many women describe increased awareness of uterine tightening, or even clearly recognizable uterine contractions over the last few days of pregnancy. With the change in production of steroids, prostaglandins, and other active agents in the placenta and fetal membranes, the stage is set for the final climactic event in pregnancy to begin. The time to be born is at hand.

Several systems must be fully functional for the birth process to start and then to proceed normally. The two most important maternal organs are the uterine muscle and the cervix. The baby is expelled from the uterus by powerful contraction of the muscle in the uterine wall. In order for the contractions of the uterus to propel the baby along the birth canal, the cervix must dilate. Throughout pregnancy the cervix has acted as a tight constriction at the opening of the uterus, helping to keep the fetus in the uterus. A popular fallacy is that the cervix is a muscle that is tightly contracted to prevent the premature departure of the baby from the uterus. The normal cervix is a tough, unyielding collection of fibrous tissue strands. The strands are made up of long thread-like molecules strongly bound to each other. Just as the many inter-woven strands of silk make silk one of the strongest fibers known, so these tightly bound fibers give the cervix great strength. The fibrous tissue of the cervix is similar to the fibrous connective tissue in a muscle tendon, or the fibers that make up the capsule of a joint such as the knee joint. The cervix contains very little muscle and is tightly closed through the whole of a normal pregnancy. Its tough structure allows the cervix to perform very well its functions of preventing the passage of the baby to the outside world before the correct time. In some pregnant women, for reasons we don't fully understand, the cervix may not be tightly closed throughout pregnancy. It may gape a little, thereby allowing the membranes that surround the fetus to bulge through into the vagina. The obstetrician may consider this an "incompetent" cervix, requiring careful watching. An incompetent cervix can lead to an early onset of labor. In cases when the cervix has a tendency to dilate early in pregnancy, the obstetrician may wish to place a stitch around the cervical canal to increase its strength.

Because the cervix is generally tightly closed, it also acts to prevent the passage of infectious agents from the vagina into the uterus. Infection is now considered a major cause of premature birth.

EN data

Fortunately in the vast majority of pregnancies, the cervix keeps tightly closed until the last three to four weeks of pregnancy when it begins to soften in preparation for dilation during the birth process. This early softening begins as a very gradual process that takes place over several days. The fibrous molecules uncurl and become less tightly adherent to each other. This softening of the cervix can often be detected by the obstetrician at a pelvic examination as early as three or four weeks before the expected date of delivery. During the early hours of delivery a striking change takes place: the cervix shortens, becomes thinner, and eventually dilates, the canal enlarging about one hundred times so that the baby can pass safely out of the uterus. Dilation of the cervix is a remarkable process in which a tight, conical structure a little bigger than the thumb becomes a floppy paper-thin structure a few millimeters thick. In the non-pregnant state and throughout the majority of pregnancy the canal in the center of the cervix is so narrow that it is hardly a canal at all. In the weeks after birth the cervix will gradually return to the shape and consistency it had before pregnancy. This reshaping of the cervix after delivery to its non-pregnant state shows that there is an amazing memory of the non-pregnant shape and consistency stored in the cells that make up the cervix. The cervix is not just an elasticized bandage that flips back into shape. The body has to actively reconstitute it in its original form.

The uterus is a muscular bag, similar in many ways to the heart. Both are beyond conscious control. There is nothing anyone can do to influence the operation of either the heart or the uterus as a conscious act of will: they are involuntary muscles. Although there are, of course, differences, the fine structure of the individual muscle cells is similar in the heart, the digestive system, and the uterus. On the other hand, uterine muscle cells are very different from the cells in muscles such as those of the limbs that can be moved voluntarily as a conscious act of will. The wall of the uterus contains two major sheets of involuntary muscle: one that is orientated in a circular fashion around the uterus and one that is placed longitudinally around the uterus. When the longitudinal muscle contracts, the uterus shortens and the fetus is driven through the cervix, providing that the cervix is adequately dilated. Contraction of both of these layers of uterine muscle is completely involuntary. A pregnant woman cannot consciously control the contraction of her uterus just as she cannot consciously control the beating of her heart or the activity of her stomach. It is this loss of active control and the fact the mother has to abandon herself to the processes of her body that makes the birth process for many women both frightening and exhilarating.

This lack of voluntary control over contraction of the uterus does not mean that the pregnant woman cannot affect the course and duration of her pregnancy by her lifestyle and various habits. There is much she can do to assure proper development of her baby and thereby lessen her risk of giving birth prematurely. Earlier in this book we discussed the effects of rest and relaxation on uterine blood flow and fetal growth and maturation. Positively developing such things as adequate exercise at a level the mother is used to, good nutrition, restful sleep, and avoiding abnormal stresses as well as unhealthy habits like tobacco, alcohol, and strong drugs, will all permit the fetus to develop his own program of events in his own way. Indeed, one can say that in most cases the fetus knows best. Left to his own devices without harmful external influences he will take care of himself very well. Eventually when he has reached a predetermined level of maturation, his next logical step is to start the birth process.

Over the last few weeks of pregnancy the body of a pregnant woman undergoes changes that are preparatory for labor. These changes in the uterus, the cervix, and the breasts occur gradually. In tissues quite distant from each other these changes have to be coordinated to take place in an orderly sequence. For example, the breast tissue has to know that it should schedule its function to be ready for breast feeding in a certain number of days. Control and coordination of these changes is choreographed by the endocrine (hormone producing) system and nervous system in conjunction with local paracrine regulators that cells use to talk to their near neighbors.

The lining of the uterus uses paracrine messages to talk to the muscle cells beneath the lining, while at the same time receiving paracrine messages from the fetal membranes that surround the fetus. With so many different conversations going on at the same time it is surprising that there is not more cross-talk! One way the body keeps the paracrine messages to cells restricted to a small region is to destroy the messenger molecules as soon as they get into the blood. In this way they can only act to influence target cells near the cells that secrete them. The whole complex interaction of nervous, endocrine, and paracrine control is like a well-trained orchestra where each player knows his role, knows just when to come in, and the intensity at which he or she is required to play. The genetic program written on the genes strung out along the chromosomes in all the fetal cells is the orchestral score from which they are all playing.

Several of these regulatory molecules alter the contractile properties of uterine muscle. As we have seen, progesterone, a steroid hormone like many of the molecules involved in the process of birth, has inhibitory effects on uterine muscle contraction. Acting in opposition to progesterone, estrogens stimulate uterine muscle contractility. They do this, in part, by instructing the lining of the uterus (the decidua) to increase the production of prostaglandins, which are paracrine regulatory compounds. The prostaglandins diffuse from cells of the decidua to the muscle cells beneath it and stimulate them to contract. The level, type, and pattern of uterine muscle contraction is determined by the balance of factors that tend to keep the uterine muscle relatively inactive and the factors that tend to stimulate activity. Maintenance of a normal pregnancy for its full duration requires the balance to be in favor of the inhibitory factors. At birth, the regulatory balance is tilted in favor of stimulation of the muscle of the uterus. At this time the muscle switches from the irregular, weak pattern of activity it has been undergoing throughout pregnancy to strong well-coordinated labor contractions. The change in circulating hormones and paracrine regulators also causes the cervix to dilate. The birth process has begun!

A question that has intrigued medical science for centuries is what signal (or signals) changes this muscle balance and initiates normal birth at the end of pregnancy. Is it the mother or the baby who decides that it is time to make the journey to the outside world? Is it the baby who says "I am mature enough to survive in the outside world?" or does the mother say "I've had enough of you now: out you go?" Who is the pilot and who is the co-pilot?

Most of the evidence with which we feel we can answer this question comes from experimental work on sheep. A skeptic might say "The information you have given is fascinating and clearly shows that the fetal lamb initiates the birth process in pregnant sheep. However," the skeptic continues, "humans are different from sheep in so many ways. How do we know that similar systems operate in the delivery of newborn human babies?" True, human physiology differs in many ways from the physiology of other animals, but it should be remembered that the delayed delivery of the human anencephalic fetus was one of the first clues to the involvement of the fetus in initiating his own delivery. That the fetus should have the ability to begin the processes that lead to his delivery at a time when he has become adequately mature, is so advantageous that it is unlikely that, once evolved, such a valuable system would be thrown away. So what happens in a sheep is unlikely to be discarded as we go up the scale of evolution toward humans.

Most of the experiments on which these findings are based were done on sheep because in outline there are many similarities between pregnancy in sheep and that in humans, as well as for the convenience that the sheep provides. Obviously there are differences between the sheep and human systems. We have some guide as to what these differences might be from work done on other primates such as monkeys and baboons, which are our nearest evolutionary relatives.

Two lines of evidence from studies in the monkey suggest that mechanisms similar to those so carefully and clearly shown in fetal sheep are also important in initiating normal birth at the end of normal pregnancy in non-human primates. In the last ten percent of the time the sheep fetus spends in the uterus, the fetal adrenal begins to secrete more and more cortisol into his blood until at delivery the concentration of cortisol in fetal blood has risen to levels twenty times the concentration present fifteen days before birth. As mentioned above, cortisol stimulates more estrogen to be produced and less progesterone by the placenta, changing the balance of factors regulating the level of contraction of the uterine muscle.

By a different route the monkey does much the same thing. The fetal monkey adrenal predominantly secretes the steroid dehydro-epiandrosterone sulfate (or DHEAS for short). DHEAS is converted to estrogen in the placenta. If we draw a graph of the rise in cortisol in the blood of the fetal sheep in the last tenth of pregnancy and superimpose on the graph the rise in DHEAS in fetal monkey blood over the same portion of pregnancy, the lines are virtually identical (see Figure 12.2). The strategy of the two species is slightly different but the end product is the same. The

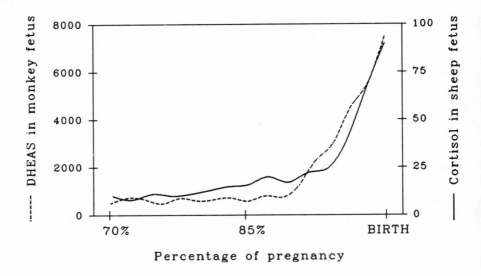

FIGURE 12.2

Comparison of the main adrenal hormone, DHEAS, in fetal monkey blood and cortisol in the fetal sheep blood in late fetal life shows the similarity in the rise in the blood concentrations of these fetal adrenal products.

fetal monkey instructs his adrenal glands to produce precursors or building blocks from which the cells in the placenta can make estrogen. The fetal sheep on the other hand uses cortisol to produce enzymes in the placenta, which convert progesterone to estrogen. In both species estrogen enhances the effect of the oxytocin, which is produced by the mother (which will be described in the next chapter), stimulating prostaglandin production and leading to an enhanced ability of the uterine muscle to contract.

The overriding point of importance is that in both species it is the fetal brain, through the mechanism of the hypothalamo-hypophyseal-adrenal axis, that plays the fundamental role in deciding the length of pregnancy. In both species it is the little guy in the uterus who is in the pilot's seat.

So the fetus is not a passive participant in the birth process after all. He actually initiates the events that result in normal birth at the end of normal pregnancy. He does this by manufacturing and secreting a cascade of blood-borne hormones and local instructional molecules. The initiating process takes place gradually over several days. As the momentum of the process increases, more and more maternal and fetal mechanisms are recruited to ensure that the process of birth moves forward in a speedy but carefully controlled fashion. Together these maternal and fetal regulatory factors stimulate the uterine muscle to contract efficiently and regularly. These same hormonal changes that stimulate contraction of uterine muscle also cause the cervix to soften. The cervix dilates to let the baby, as Hippocrates said, "Burst forth into the world, free of all bonds."

Chapter 13

Labor and Delivery: A Job for Two

Birth is too important a process to be regulated by a single mechanism. If a single mechanism were responsible for labor, and if that mechanism failed, the baby and the mother would be at risk. Once the birth process begins it must be completed in a timely fashion. To achieve a smooth, escalating process, a cascade of mechanisms is rapidly brought into play. Some of the processes are controlled by the mother and some by the fetus. The final act of labor is a collaboration between them both. The existence of many back-ups and fail-safe mechanisms helps to explain why the vast majority of deliveries proceed smoothly without problems.

Several hormones are involved in labor and delivery. As described in the last chapter, estrogens stimulate production of a group of paracrine regulatory molecules (prostaglandins), which stimulate strong contractions of the uterine muscle. They are produced in the fetal membranes, in the placenta, in the lining of the uterus, and by the uterine muscle cells. During pregnancy, one of the actions of progesterone is to inhibit the production of prostaglandins, thereby keeping to a minimum any tendency for the uterus to begin labor and delivery contractions. In their turn, prostaglandins are able to inhibit progesterone production. Once progesterone production begins to decrease, more and more prostaglandins are produced, beginning an escalating "positive feed forward" system.

Positive feed forward systems are self-potentiating: they gain power from their own momentum once they get started. The purpose of the positive feed forward system brought into play in the birth process is gradually and inexorably to accelerate and intensify the whole process of birth. Positive feed forward systems get things done quickly, but at a price. They are very difficult to control. They are potentially very dangerous because they just keep increasing and increasing—rather like a runaway nuclear reactor. Positive feed forward is used sparingly by the body and only at exceptional times. It is really only safe when a process has a natural termination that must be achieved in a limited time. The birth of a baby is just such a case. After all, once the baby is out of the uterus and the placenta has delivered, that is the end of the process. The stretching of the uterus by its contents that stimulates contraction, the stimulus to production of estrogen by the placenta, and the production of prostaglandins no longer occur. So positive feed forward is acceptable, even desirable, in processes that result in their own termination. It brings the event to a more rapid conclusion.

In contrast, a negative feedback system works in just the opposite way. An example can be seen in the way we control our blood pressure. If anything happens to raise blood pressure significantly, little sensors in the arteries send messages to the brain saying "Blood pressure going up, take remedial action!" The remedial action involves several changes, including slowing the rate and strength at which the heart beats. As a result pressure in the blood circulatory system falls until the normal range is reached again. Negative feedback systems are designed to achieve long-term stability within a narrow range of function.

Prostaglandins, which we have already seen are paracrine (local regulatory molecules), in addition to inhibiting progesterone production, act directly on the muscle of the uterus to cause it to contract. Prostaglandins also cause softening of the cervix, which helps the cervix to dilate. Regulatory compounds can affect more

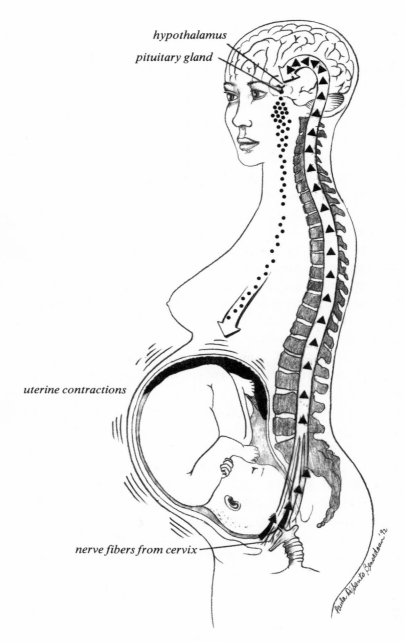

FIGURE 13.1

Reflexive release of oxytocin. Nerve fibers from the cervix carry messages to the mother's brain to stimulate the release of oxytocin. Oxytocin then stimulates uterine contraction.

than one system, pulling together more and more components of the complex interactive process. The birth process begins inexorably to build in response to hormones that have multiple actions into a full-speed-ahead positive feed forward.

Once the process of delivery has begun, many factors are recruited to increase the strength of uterine contractions. A major contribution by the mother is oxytocin, a powerful hormone secreted from the maternal pituitary gland. Oxytocin is released into the mother's blood and stimulates the muscle cells in the uterus to contract strongly. As a result of the contractions, the cervix is stretched. The cervix is also stretched by the baby's head as labor progresses and this stimulates the release of more oxytocin from the mother's pituitary gland by way of a nervous reflex. Nerve fibers carry impulses from the cervix up the mother's spinal cord to her brain. The reflexive release of oxytocin by the mother in turn causes further uterine contraction. Likewise, this uterine contraction in its turn stimulates more oxytocin release. This loop that regulates maternal oxytocin secretion is an excellent example of positive feed forward.

Oxytocin has another action that speeds along the labor process. It also stimulates the release of prostaglandins from the maternal cells that line the uterine cavity. The released prostaglandins stimulate the uterine muscle to contract ever more strongly. With both of these powerful stimulators of uterine muscle contraction, oxytocin and prostaglandins, being produced by systems that employ positive feed forward, it is no surprise that it is very difficult to stop labor once it has started. So we can see that the normal birth process involves nervous, endocrine, and paracrine factors. This set of processes with its many participants contains interconnected positive feed forward loops that interact in a carefully programmed sequence.

The birth process brings into play all the marvelous response mechanisms the fetus has matured during the last few weeks of pregnancy. Constant squeezing by the uterus results in pressure on the fetal head during its passage down the birth canal. This stimulates the fetus to release thyroid hormones and adrenaline that will assist him to regulate his temperature when he is in the outside world. The pressure on his head will also help to prevent him from taking any breaths until his head has completely emerged from of the birth canal. It is very important that he should not try to breathe because he might inhale fluids from the birth canal. He waits to breathe until his head is out. Then he can breathe air safely.

The margin of safety that nature allows the baby in the birth process is more than adequate. Studies in lambs have clearly shown that the oxygen levels in the fetal lamb's blood fall only a little, if at all, during a normal birth. All these beautiful compensatory mechanisms for maintaining oxygen supply to the brain continue to function amazingly efficiently during delivery. In addition, the obstetrician can monitor the fetal heart beat to ensure that the fetus is in good condition and coping well with the challenges of birth. Mothers can be reassured that the human baby has developed remarkable strategies to cope with the whole process of being born. In fact, the problems he faces are generally far fewer than those facing the tenth puppy or piglet in a litter. With correct preparation and attention to health needs throughout pregnancy, the process of delivery is generally a very natural process if pregnancy goes to the normal full term. Indeed, there are indications that the many stresses that result from vaginal delivery are actually good for the baby, that he is generally better prepared for extrauterine life than a baby delivered by cesarean section. Delivery by cesarean section short-circuits the process of preparation for life outside the uterus, avoiding the repeated episodes of stimulation provided by contractions. Only future research will tell us the implications each of these routes of delivery has on future development of the newborn baby and possibly into adult life.

It would appear then, that contractions serve a wider function than simply propelling the baby out through the cervix, and are not without their own medical mystery. They are an obvious and uncomfortable feature of the birth process. Contractions are generally short, lasting not much more than a minute, and occur every few minutes or so. They are well coordinated and efficient. Earlier in pregnancy, however, there are repeated bouts of activity of the uterine muscle that are less apparent, lasting five to fifteen minutes and occurring every twenty to forty minutes. We have

A

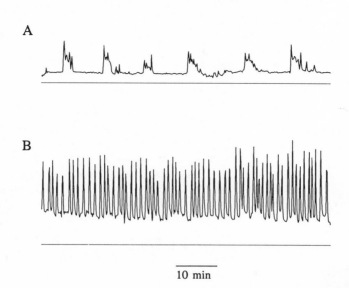

B

10 min

FIGURE 13.2

Two types of uterine muscle activity patterns exist during pregnancy. (A) The pressure changes produced by contractures that occur throughout pregnancy, and (B) during labor contractions.

named these low grade bouts of uterine contractility *contractures*, to distinguish them from contractions.

Contractures are a form of uterine activity that occurs throughout the majority of pregnancy in every species so far studied, including monkeys and baboons. We are reasonably confident that it is possible to build a picture of what happens to pregnant women. The only way of monitoring human pregnancy for contractile activity is with the tocodynamometer, which is strapped to the woman's abdomen. This little gadget is reasonably useful if the woman is very slim. More than thirty pounds of excess body fat when pregnant renders the readings unreliable. Medical science is urgently in need of a diagnostic machine equivalent to the electrocardiogram (EKG) to be used in pregnancy. The EKG gives very precise readings of human heart activity. Unfortunately, the obstetricians do not have such a machine to track the contraction

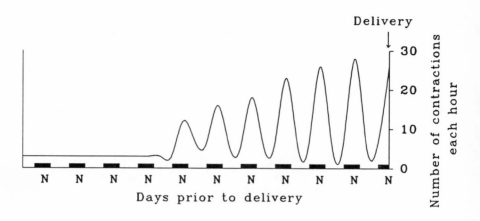

FIGURE 13.3
Nightly bursts of contraction activity over several nights before delivery as recorded from a pregnant monkey. N is night-time.

of the uterus. If they did they would be much better able to identify normal and abnormal labor.

In 1872, a physician named John Braxton Hicks drew attention to the fact that many women feel a tightening in the abdomen at fairly frequent intervals during pregnancy. When a woman describes them they sound remarkably like the contractures recorded in experimental studies in animals. Braxton Hicks' contractions are by no means common to all women. Some women experience an entire pregnancy without reporting feeling any Braxton Hicks' contractions. Without adequately sensitive recording devices we can only suppose that contractures in many women are below the level of sensation that they can feel. Many women do not even feel fairly strong contractions that can be recorded by the toco-dynamometer—just as many women do not feel all of the movements of the fetus that can be observed during an ultrasound scan.

At the time of birth, contractures change to contractions. This switch is essential if normal safe expulsion of the baby is to occur. A better understanding of the mechanisms that underlie this switch from contractures to contractions would greatly improve our ability to anticipate, diagnose, and prevent premature birth. More research and better instrumentation are needed to define the normal patterns of activity and to identify the factors and situations in which contractures change to contractions.

One area of enquiry that may hold answers to many questions is discovering the role that the mother's twenty-four-hour clock may play in the precise regulation of the time of the day or night the baby is born.

In pregnant monkeys maintained in an environment in which the lighting is precisely controlled so that lights are on for fourteen hours each day and off for ten hours, the switch from contractures to contractions is related to the onset of darkness. It is a very dramatic switch. One moment the pattern of uterine activity is of the contracture pattern that has been occurring through most of the pregnancy. The next moment uterine activity consists only of contractions, indicating the onset of labor.

Labor and delivery contraction activity seems to develop progressively over several days. A characteristic feature of normal delivery in the monkey is the observation that on the first evening after the switch from contractures to contractions occurs, the contractions only last an hour or so. The contractions then revert to contractures. On the next night contractures again switch to contractions, and the period of contraction activity usually lasts a little longer and the force of the individual contractions is a little stronger than the first night of the switch. On subsequent nights the duration of the period of contractions increases until eventually on one night contractions continue until the baby is born. Although the contractions begin around the time the lights go out, the actual timing of day or night the baby is delivered will depend on the length of the labor necessary for the baby to be delivered. The length of the labor will depend on many factors such as the size of the baby relative to the size of the mother, the strength of the contractions, proper dilation of the cervix, and the mother's ability to push voluntarily with her abdominal muscles.

The recurring period of contraction activity for several nights before birth occurs is described by many pregnant women. I have my own family anecdote. On a recent visit to my hometown I sat down for a cup of tea with a young niece, Alison. Three days earlier

Alison had delivered her second baby, young Callum who was sleeping in his crib faithfully attended by his three-year-old sister Charlotte. "How was the birth?" I asked Alison. "Peter, it was so strange," she replied "I must have gone into labor every night for a week." At this point I stopped her. Knowing the skepticism of my scientific colleagues I asked Alison to be prepared to confirm that I had not, and did not intend to, lead the witness in her description of Callum's birth. I asked her to be prepared to give me a notarized confirmation that the description of Callum's birth was hers alone, without prompting or interference from me. She laughed, I think sensing what was in my mind.

Part of the relevance of this story is that Alison, in her mid-twenties, is an accountant who hates hospitals. She is completely non-medical. She is very disturbed by the smell of ether or anything to do with biology and medical science. She was certainly not on the look-out for points of medical interest, and certainly not about to support my hypothesis.

"Every night for a week before Callum was born," Alison continued, "I felt a lot of tightening around dinner time. I knew it wasn't real labor. The pains weren't like the labor pains I had when Charlotte was born. Then after six or seven evenings, late on Tuesday evening (three days prior to our conversation) I knew I was going to deliver that night. Malcolm and I got into our car, went to the hospital, and Callum was born about one in the morning."

"You are describing exactly what happens when pregnant monkeys go into labor," I now felt able to say. "They have activity for several nights before they deliver." "I'm not a monkey" Alison interjected amid general laughter, which put an end to any serious consideration of biological kinship and what we could learn from experimental science by comparing labor in pregnant women with that of monkeys. "That's what you think," I thought to myself, making a note of what she had said.

If only we knew the factors responsible for this twenty-four-hour rhythm with a recurring peak of contraction activity in the early hours of the night, our understanding of normal birth as well as premature birth would be greatly enhanced. The concentrations of several key hormones in the blood of both fetus and mother show clear twenty-four-hour rhythms in the concentration of estrogens and their precursor DHEAS. These pronounced twenty-four-hour rhythms undoubtedly in some way influence the switch of uterine muscle contractile activity from contractures to contractions.

It is important, however, to distinguish the factors that set the scene and initiate the preparatory changes for labor and delivery in both the uterus and cervix, from those factors that precisely set the time of the day at which the baby is born. If the physician allows the pregnancy to run its normal course, human births occur more frequently at night-time. Experimental evidence also suggests that maternal factors have considerable control over the final timing of birth. The nature of this control of the precise time of the day or night the baby is born is not well understood. It is probably not a conscious mechanism, although the contractile patterns of labor and delivery may be influenced by stress in some animals, such as pregnant mares. If strangers are present, pregnant mares are able to exercise some control over the final timing of delivery. They are very easily stressed by the presence of strangers. You may have tried to watch the foaling of a mare to whom you were a stranger. You may have stayed around for hours awaiting the pleasure of seeing the foal's entry into the world. If your patience lapsed and you retired for just a few minutes to get a cup of tea, you probably found on return that the foal had been born. You may have thought the mare just ornery. Well, she wasn't: she was just stressed by your presence, and refused to complete the process while you were there. If the cervix is fully open, the final stages of delivery depend very much on contraction of maternal abdominal muscles as opposed to the uterine muscle. The abdominal muscles can be voluntarily controlled by the mare.

The fetus did his bit by starting off the increased synthesis of estrogen many days earlier. It appears that the role of estrogens is to raise the level of irritability and responsiveness of the uterine muscle cell to enable it to contract when another signal appears, which probably comes from the mother. Thus, although the fetus decides when pregnancy has lasted long enough and that he is mature enough and initiates the whole process of delivery, the mother finally has to be ready as well. She determines the time of day at which labor begins.

Maternal control over the time of day at which delivery occurs is of biological value insofar as the mother can deliver the baby at a safe time of the day. Some animals tend to choose a time when predators are absent or optimal climatic conditions exist. Rats, for example, are normally active at night, and during the day, the pregnant female rat is generally safely in the nest. Usually they deliver in the afternoon, during the daylight hours. Pregnant alpacas high in the altiplano of the South American Andes deliver their young in the early hours of the morning. Thus, the young are not exposed immediately after birth to the brutally cold Andean nights, but have time to become dry and mobile. Pregnant women tend to deliver during the night-time. Most primates are daytime-active animals, and at night they are safely within the confines of whatever home or resting place they have. It may not be a coincidence that the Christmas story takes place at night with a special star overhead.

Although we now know that the fetus determines the overall duration of pregnancy making the decision to start the birth process, the maternal systems are predominant in the control of the precise timing of delivery. There are as many questions still to be answered as there are those of which we have some understanding. That the precise timing of birth is related in some way to the night/day clock is clear. Until we have better technology to use in our experimental studies we have our noses up against the window of knowledge, peering into the unknown.

Chapter 14

NEWBORN ADAPTATION TO LIFE

We cry that we are come to this great stage of fools.
William Shakespeare, *King Lear*

King Lear was right to think of birth as a dramatic, indeed theatrical entrance to the world stage. His reference to "fools" also has a certain poignancy in light of what has been said about the tragic and avoidable consequences of substance abuse. He was, of course, medically quite wrong in thinking that a baby cries at birth because he suddenly realizes what he has let himself in for.

What actually happens, and the reason for the cry, is that toward the end of the passage of the baby's head through the birth canal, short-lived, mild hypoxemia generally occurs. The margin of safety in oxygen delivery to the fetus, and his ability to extract more oxygen from his blood in times of minor oxygen shortage, means that this degree of oxygen lack is natural and not life-threatening. This decrease in fetal oxygen is the result of several events that are happening simultaneously. The muscle in the wall of the uterus is contracting strongly. Each contraction squeezes the maternal blood vessels as they go through the wall of the uterus to the placenta. As a result, less maternal blood passes through the wall to the placenta. Thus, less oxygen is delivered to the maternal side of the placenta. The umbilical cord, the fetal life-line that contains the blood vessels that connect him to the placenta, is being stretched, and even possibly squashed, by the contractions. Finally the placenta begins to separate from the wall of the uterus. Despite these changes the baby generally does not make his first attempt to breathe until his head is out of the birth canal. It may well be that the fetal paradoxical response to hypoxemia is still operating and his brain tells him not to breathe in response to hypoxemia quite yet—that need will come soon.

An additional control mechanism is also telling him not to breathe. During labor, prostaglandin production by the placenta increases. The concentration of prostaglandins rises in the fetal as well as the maternal blood. Experimental studies have shown that increasing prostaglandin concentrations in the blood of a fetal sheep will inhibit his breathing efforts. Conversely, inhibiting the production of prostaglandins will stimulate breathing. Here we see the beautiful efficiency and economy of design that have been demonstrated at all stages of fetal life. The very processes that are fundamental in bringing about the process of delivery also act to ensure that the fetus does not put himself at risk by breathing during the birth process. Again we see how wonderfully inter-connected are the various fetal, placental, and maternal systems. The several processes occurring at labor are so well orchestrated that prostaglandins, one of the major factors helping to propel the fetus into the outside world, also play a role in stopping him from breathing. It is very important that the baby doesn't breathe during the birth process. If he does try to breathe while his head is in the birth canal, he may well inhale blood and other fluids into his lungs, thereby risking the development of pneumonia.

When the baby's head exits from the birth canal he meets the outside world for the first time. In this new world many things are changed forever. When the umbilical cord is tied off, the source of production of prostaglandins from the placenta is removed and the passage of prostaglandins into the baby's circulation ceases immediately. The prostaglandins circulating in his blood disappear in a very few minutes. Thus, one of the major factors inhibiting his breathing is removed and he is free to breathe naturally if other stimuli to his brain instruct him to do so. The temperature of his new world is colder than he has experienced during his life so far.

The release of the pressure on his head and other sensory stimuli combine with an altered response to hypoxemia to stimulate his respiratory center in his brain, instructing him to take that important first breath. His cry announces to the world "I am here."

We have seen that even while he was a fetus, the baby's brain was very good at controlling his reactions to situations such as hypoxemia. Now at the time of birth the newborn baby's brain takes control completely. A major reorganization takes place in the way his brain controls his breathing patterns. Remember, the paradoxical fetal response to low oxygen availability resulted in the fetus stopping breathing whenever he became short of oxygen. That is the last thing the newborn baby must do, so the brain must totally reorganize the way it responds to oxygen deficiency. It used to be thought that the switch from the paradoxical response to hypoxemia to increased breathing in response to hypoxemia was sudden and complete at birth. Studies with newborn animals show that in many species the transition between these two opposite responses is not quite as clear or quick as previously thought. Newborn lambs respond to oxygen deprivation by an initial increase in breathing, but they cannot maintain high rates of breathing in response to the hypoxemia. Although their breathing rate remains elevated, they can only maintain this increased rate at the maximal level for a few minutes. As has been described, studies such as those investigating the newborn lamb's response to hypoxemia will eventually help pediatricians to develop methods that will alert parents of babies who might be at risk for SIDS. It is very likely that in the next few years researchers will be able to devise tests to detect the babies who are at risk. Much more research needs to be done.

Birth is a time of great challenge to the newborn baby's body systems. All the preparation that has been taking place in late fetal life is now rapidly put to the test. No longer does the baby's heart need to pump blood to the placenta. Bypassing the lungs by the shunting blood through the ductus arteriosus and foramen ovale in the heart must be stopped, at once. Systems and strategies that were appropriate for him as a fetus in the uterus are no longer appropriate for an independent newborn baby.

The first breath is a vital, assertive, and independent act. It has been said that we achieve no greater feat in the whole of our lives than we do with our first breath. To some extent this dramatic statement has to be true. If we do not accomplish our first breath successfully, we will not accomplish anything. Four critical changes take place simultaneously as a direct result of the first breath. The lungs are ventilated with air containing oxygen; the flap over the foramen ovale closes; the umbilical cord is stretched and the umbilical arteries close down, cutting off the fetal circulation to the placenta; and the ductus arteriosus closes down. Let us look at the causes and consequences of each of these critical events.

With the first and subsequent breaths, air is drawn into the lungs and, providing the lung is adequately mature, the air sacs open. The oxygen in the air has a direct relaxing effect on the muscle walls of the blood vessels in the baby's lungs causing these vessels to dilate. The resistance to blood flow in the lungs now falls rapidly and blood flows through the pulmonary artery into the lungs rather than across the ductus arteriosus and into the aorta. This blood is oxygenated as it passes through the lungs. It then returns via the pulmonary veins into the left atrium of the heart. Suddenly, there is a large increase in the amount of blood returning to the left atrium and as a result the pressure in the left atrium increases. The left atrial pressure now exceeds the right atrial pressure for the first time and the small flap valve on the left side of the septum between the two atria is pushed against the septum. The flow of blood through the foramen ovale is shut off at once. This flap valve was previously kept open because the pressure in the right atrium was greater than that in the left atrium. So one of the fetal shunts, the foramen ovale, closes immediately. If all is well, blood no longer passes from the right atrium to the left atrium.

Over the next few weeks, the margins of the flap over the foramen ovale are joined tightly to the rest of the wall between the right and left atrium by the ingrowth of a dense network of fibrous tissue. The result is permanent structural closure of the foramen ovale. If there is a deficiency in the flap, or the hole is too large to close, a persistent pathway may remain. If the foramen ovale stays open the baby is said to have a type of hole in the heart. Depending on the size of the hole and the amount of blood that passes through it, special surgery may be required to close the flap. Because the pressure gradient across the wall between the two atria is now from left to right, any blood that does continue to flow through the foramen ovale will just go around the lungs twice. While this double circuit is inefficient, it is not as life-threatening as the situation in which the blood bypasses the lungs completely.

The umbilical arteries are very sensitive to stretching. As the baby is delivered the umbilical cord stretches and the umbilical arteries automatically clamp down very firmly. If they did not, the baby would be in danger of losing much blood when the umbilical cord eventually breaks. Of course, in attended deliveries the umbilical cord is tied as a precaution. Both the stretching and tying of the umbilical cord have the same effect. They raise the pressure in the systemic circulation because the newborn baby's blood system is no longer connected to the low placental resistance.

So two major changes have occurred in the circulatory system. The resistance on the left side of the circulation has increased and the resistance in the pulmonary circulation has fallen dramatically as the lungs open up and breathing begins. The increased pressure in the aorta now exceeds the pressure in the pulmonary artery and blood begins to flow in the opposite direction through the ductus arteriosus, flowing now from the aorta through to the pulmonary artery. This blood in the aorta has come from the left ventricle having just been through the lungs, and it is, therefore, well oxygenated. Oxygen stimulates the smooth muscle cells in the wall of the ductus arteriosus to contract thereby shutting it off. This shutdown takes a few hours and during that time the pediatrician may hear a murmur over the baby's heart. This murmur, like many others in the newborn, is nothing to worry about. It just represents a little blood flowing through the ductus arteriosus in a left to right direction. The turbulent blood flow is an example of the many exciting changes going on in the newborn baby's body.

The beautiful organization of the regulation of bodily function is well illustrated by the different effects of oxygen on blood vessels in the lung when compared with the ductus arteriosus. In the lung, oxygen causes the smooth muscle cells in the walls of the blood vessels to relax. This system is designed to allow oxygen to get into the blood as it makes sense for the blood to flow to oxygen-rich areas of the lung. In contrast, oxygen causes the smooth muscle cells in the wall of the ductus arteriosus to constrict. In the oxygen-rich world outside the uterus the newborn baby will obtain his oxygen from his lungs not his placenta, so the body uses oxygen as a signal to shut off the bypass that shunts blood away from the lungs to the placenta. The newborn baby doesn't have a placenta anyway! It has been thrown away as surplus to requirement. It is truly a miracle how oxygen instructs one set of muscles in the walls of one set of blood vessels to relax, and another set of muscle cells in different vessels to contract.

During fetal life, prostaglandins in the fetal blood acted to relax the muscle in the ductus arteriosus thus helping to keep it open. Now as the prostaglandins disappear from the newborn baby's blood and oxygen concentrations in the blood rise, the ductus muscle contracts and cuts off the blood flowing through it. In a few hours it has completely shut down and the shunt between the pulmonary artery and aorta is finally closed. Until the ductus arteriosus finally closes the pressure gradient dictates that any flow is in the direction of left to right. This is not a great threat to the newborn baby as flow from aorta to pulmonary artery just results in a second passage of a relatively small amount of blood through the lungs without going to the tissues all around the body first. With any small left to right passage of blood through the foramen ovale, this second passage through the lungs is a little inefficient, but unless the flow through the shunt is high, there is no great extra strain on the heart. Eventually, the closure of the ductus arteriosus becomes permanent when the ductus tissues are invaded by cells that produce a dense web of fibers that obliterate the central core of the blood vessel.

As a result of these changes in the circulation, the newborn baby can now provide himself with oxygen from his lungs (as long as they have matured correctly). The two shunts have been closed and the pressure has changed dramatically in several parts of the circulation. If the lung is immature and the air sacs cannot be maintained open, oxygenation will be inadequate. In this situation the newborn baby is at considerable risk. If the pulmonary blood vessels remain closed and pulmonary resistance remains high, the foramen ovale and ductus arteriosus may remain open and blood will continue to bypass the lungs. It is as if the newborn baby is saying to himself "My lungs are not functioning well, so I will bypass my lungs, and send my blood through the foramen ovale and ductus arteriosus to the placenta. After all, that course of action has worked throughout my life in the uterus." Unfortunately there is no longer a functional placenta, so bypassing the lungs has no benefit and indeed makes the situation even worse. The neonatologist treating newborn babies suffering from respiratory problems must work hard to maintain adequate oxygenation, correct the direction of blood flow through the shunts to the normal newborn state, and thereby eventually produce their permanent closure.

Precise information on the regulation of fetal and neonatal breathing movements has been obtained by painstaking research over many years. As has been shown, surfactant, a group of fatty molecules that lower the surface tension in the air sacs of the baby's lung, is very important. Carefully designed studies have increased our understanding of the role of surfactant in lowering the surface tension of the air sacs of the lung and the control of its production by the fetus' own hormones. Such studies have also improved our knowledge of the factors that regulate blood flow through the fetal and newborn lung. The information obtained has been vital for developing clinical management procedures used in the neonatal intensive care unit. Thousands of small premature babies owe their lives to the implementation of knowledge derived from animal experimentation.

As a direct result, and as if to show that knowledge knows no boundaries, the management procedures developed in the human neonatal intensive care unit are now being used for the treatment of premature animals, especially premature foals. In one respect we may say that the premature foal is beginning to benefit from two decades of information gained by managing newborn babies. The newborn human baby has been an experimental animal model for the newborn foal.

We have seen that cortisol secreted by the fetus himself plays a key role in bringing about the increase in surfactant production that precedes birth at the end of a pregnancy of normal duration. Cortisol also prepares the thyroid system for the increased activity that is necessary so that the newborn can increase his heat production in response to the colder temperature outside the uterus. Many other key newborn capabilities are the result of the action of fetal cortisol on the tissues of the fetal body in the last days of life before birth.

Cortisol is also the link the fetus uses between his brain and the placenta to commence the birth process (see Chapter 12). The linkage of the maturation of key organ systems to the same mechanisms that initiate birth is the way the fetus tries to ensure that when he is born, his vital systems will all be completely prepared for the transition to the outside world. Unfortunately, as we shall see in the next chapter, birth occurs prematurely in about one in ten of all pregnancies in the developed countries. The rate is higher in developing countries. There are many causes of premature birth. In all instances the prematurely born baby is at considerable risk. The extent of the risk depends on how far along the normal developmental path his various body systems, especially his lungs, have progressed by the time he is born and must depend on them.

After birth the newborn baby's brain begins to receive a flood of information that differs from the input it received during life before birth. He is now living in an atmosphere that contains five times as much oxygen as was available when he was a fetus. The higher oxygen concentrations significantly change the opportunities for the newborn; his nerve cells are now able to work at a higher rate and to develop the full range of their capabilities.

In addition to incorporating the new sensory input, the newborn baby must adjust his behavior to that of his mother to obtain the optimal nutrition by feeding at the breast. In all mammals, bonding between mother and infant is of critical importance to a lasting relationship, and hence proper development of the baby.

There are several interesting studies of newborn and infant behavior that show how critical the environment is to the development of the baby's brain. The key to our success as a species is the combination of parental care and the extraordinary capacity of the human newborn nervous system to receive, assimilate, and organize information. Our brains are insatiable storage organs that develop capacities in proportion to how much they are used when they are young and responsive. As has been seen in the chapter on the brain, several experimental studies have shown that the ability of nerve cells to develop connections with neighboring cells is improved with activity. Young animals reared in an exciting, challenging environment with plentiful and varied sensory input develop a more capable nervous system.

Adaptation to the outside world means that the newborn baby must now look to balance his own fluid and mineral intake and output. Before birth the placenta acted as a fetal kidney. Water and the various salts that make up our internal body fluids were transported across the placenta as needed. From experimental studies we know a great deal about transport across the placenta in sheep (Chapter 5), but very little about the regulation of placental transport of these vitally important body components across the human placenta. Generally, when the placenta is functioning normally, the fetus does not suffer from deficiency or excess of any important constituent of his body fluids. Indeed, exquisitely sensitive mechanisms have been developed by the fetus and placenta to maintain the internal fetal environment. An excellent example is how the placenta regulates the availability of calcium, a major component of every cell in the body. Calcium is vital to normal bone formation as well as to the secretory processes of all cells. Studies have shown that a fetal sheep maintains a normal blood calcium level regardless of whether his mother eats a normal, very high or deficient calcium diet. The placenta regulates the passage of calcium from mother to fetus, increasing transfer of calcium to the fetus in times of maternal calcium shortage, and decreasing calcium transport to the fetus in times of maternal calcium excess. This protective ability of the placenta is vital to the production of normal bones for the baby.

After birth, calcium and all other food components are delivered in the milk into the newborn baby's digestive system. The digestive system is far less able than was the placenta to adjust intake, and the composition of the baby's bodily fluids is controlled by regulating loss through the kidneys. The kidneys of the newborn baby are not fully developed. One function that still needs to improve is the ability of the kidney to excrete water should the newborn drink too much fluid. We should remember that his mother's milk is the most appropriate form of fluid for the newborn baby, both in quantity of constituents as well as their relative proportions.

The neonatal period is one of intense excitement for parents, the extended family, and friends. Babies learn new feats each day; new cries, new movements, new smiles. Their nutritional demands increase as they grow and develop. The period of parental care provided for the newborn human is the longest of any animal species. Babies' interactions with their environment cement the bond between the baby and parents, and at the same time provide their developing central nervous system with input that is vital to their development.

The knowledge we have acquired about life before birth can help us to understand the newborn baby's needs. We shall see in the next chapter how vital this information has been in assisting pediatricians when things go wrong and the baby is born prematurely and has to be maintained in a neonatal intensive care unit (NICU). Even the baby born at the end of a completely normal pregnancy benefits from a better understanding of the factors that have controlled his development and those that will operate in the early days, weeks, and months of life after birth.

Let us take as an example the question of rest and wakefulness in the newborn. As we have seen, the sensory information pouring into the fetal brain is not just absorbed and stored but also affects the development of the brain. Just as you or I do not like to be disturbed at certain times and respond well at others, so the baby's brain will respond differently at various times of the day. Much more systematic and controlled research needs to be conducted before we know what strategies we should adopt to improve fetal brain development, both in at-risk fetuses as well as normal fetuses; the same applies to newborn babies born at the end of a normal pregnancy as it does to those born prematurely. Current knowledge places us firmly on the threshold of an era in which we will be able to suggest rational and efficacious therapies to be coordinated in the NICU. These strategies must be based on firm knowledge of fetal life. Life before birth has provided the baby with all the systems necessary for him to develop to his full potential. He is now ready for the future.

Chapter 15

PREMATURITY:
BORN TOO SOON OR TOO SMALL

I, that am curtail'd of this fair proportion cheated of feature by dissembling nature, Deform'd unfinish'd, sent before my time into this breathing world, scarce half made up.
William Shakespeare, *Richard III*

A premature baby is one who is born before he has had a chance to fully program the development of all his organ systems so that they are ready to function outside the life-support system of the mother's uterus. We have seen how the fetus works from an internal blueprint: he has a program of carefully orchestrated developmental events designed to ensure adequate development of lung, digestive system, muscle, and bone by the time he is born, and we have seen how at all times he prioritizes the development of his brain. The process is so well designed that normal birth uses the same signal systems that were necessary for the development of vital organs such as lungs. The processes of birth and maturation are closely linked together. This linkage helps to prevent a mismatch caused by the birth of a baby who is too immature to survive outside the uterus.

Unfortunately, sometimes things go wrong and the baby is born prematurely, before he is fully ready for the next stage of his great adventure. Let us look at the common causes of premature birth and look at the consequences of being "born before one's time." Babies born before thirty-seven weeks of pregnancy are considered premature. However, the date of the last menstrual period is not always accurately known, so whether a baby is classified as premature is often decided on the baby's birth weight. According to the birth weight system, a baby less than twenty-five hundred grams (three-and-a-half pounds) is considered premature. Another method of classification is to consider all babies under twenty-five hundred grams as low birth weight. Babies less than fifteen hundred grams (about one percent of all babies born) are described as very low birth weight. Two out of every thousand babies are extremely low birth weight babies weighing less than seven hundred fifty grams.

The incidence of premature birth in the United States is just under ten percent. At least seventy-five percent of fetal death during labor or in the first month of the baby's life is associated with premature birth. Low birth weight babies are two hundred times more likely to die in the first year of life. Premature babies are also ten times more likely to suffer from a major neurological handicap than babies born after the full length of pregnancy. They are more susceptible to long-term problems that will impair their lives, such as visual disturbances and impaired lung function. Sixteen percent of very low birth weight babies and thirty percent of extremely low birth weight babies will have lasting neurological impairment.

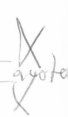

Establishing the causes of premature birth has not been easy. Until recently, the vast bulk of evidence was obtained from statistical analysis of medical records. We are right to be wary of statistics, but they can often yield important clues. There are several conditions that are known to be associated with premature labor. We must remember that a statistical association between two events is just that—an association. The association of two events in time does not prove a causal effect. Epidemiology is the science of association of disease conditions with environmental and family history, lifestyle, and other factors that may play a role in a disease. Epidemiology is a powerful discipline but it can only point the way to causal links.

One of the major achievements of epidemiology was the linkage of tobacco smoke to lung cancer in the 1960s. The linkage is very firm, yet the tobacco industry is still able to deny any causal relationship because epidemiology lacks the ability of the scientific experimental study to show incontrovertible evidence that when we change just one factor, something else inevitably happens. This is the only reliable way to show cause and effect.

As an example of scientific study, if we remove the pancreas from a rat, the rat will become diabetic. It is not necessary to remove the pancreas surgically. There are drugs that will destroy the cells in the pancreas that produce insulin. These drugs cause diabetes. For additional evidence, one can see under a microscope that it is only the cells of the pancreas that produce insulin, which are killed by the drugs. Other cells in the pancreas are not destroyed. The final proof that the diabetes is caused by lack of insulin can be provided by injecting insulin and reversing the effects of removal of the pancreas.

I have dwelt on this example to emphasize the need for controlled scientific experiments in the search for the causes of prematurity. Epidemiological evidence provides enormously valuable information, but by itself it does not prove cause and effect. Cigarette smoking increased rapidly during and following the First World War in which bored soldiers sat in their muddy trenches with nothing to do for hours on end but smoke and await the inevitable bayonet charge. Then, many years after the war, the incidence of lung cancer rose. For many of the heavy smokers the approach of death by lung cancer was as inevitable as the death in the trenches. Because of social factors, women began smoking later than men, and sure enough the incidence of lung cancer in women rose later than in men.

However, this association of two events was not a carefully designed experiment in which nothing else was changing. It has been said facetiously that in the years during which the cancerous tumor cells were growing in the lungs preparing to kill millions, the consumption of bananas was also rising. So, it could be argued, from the point of view of just association in time, that the banana was just as likely to be a cause of lung cancer as was tobacco smoke. It is for reasons such as these that, while they complement each other, epidemiological association can never take the place of basic research.

Epidemiological studies can help us by showing that changing a particular feature of lifestyle or environment can decrease the incidence of a certain condition. When the first statistics appeared on the relationship of lung cancer and smoking, there was a group of professionals who quickly accepted this evidence of cause and effect. These were the physicians who had to treat the unfortunate sufferers who had lung cancer following years of heavy smoking. Many of these physicians stopped smoking. As a result they unconsciously provided a study that could help us determine cause and effect. What happened was that the incidence of cancer dropped in the physicians who had given up smoking, while those who continued to smoke continued to succumb to the disease in large numbers. Even this clear-cut study could be challenged, and was discounted by the tobacco industry as only showing that the disease rate dropped in those who had the will-power to give up smoking, suggesting that those physicians with 'will-power' were a separate group and other factors in this group might have influenced the disease.

Much has been learned about prematurity from epidemiological studies. We now know that there are certain maternal conditions that put the mother at risk to have a premature baby. Prematurity is more common in very young women and in women who are pregnant at the end of their child-bearing years. There is also a higher tendency for premature birth associated with previous premature births, with certain maternal illnesses such as kidney disease, and fibroids and other structural abnormalities in the uterus. It is easy to see how structural abnormalities may result in early rupture of the membranes or lack of an adequate surface of the uterine lining for the placenta to perform effectively. The possibility of diagnosing and improving these conditions is high if obstetrician and mother-to-be get together for proper prenatal care throughout pregnancy.

As we have seen, one epidemiological study showed that women who were themselves growth-retarded at birth run a greater risk of having a premature delivery. The mechanisms that are responsible for this association of a mother's own birth history and that of her child are far from clear. Sometimes it is easy to see why a particular pregnancy ends in premature delivery. For instance, excessive production of amniotic fluid (polyhydramnios) stretches the uterus more than usual. The response of any muscle when stretched is to contract. If this tendency becomes pronounced due to increasing polyhydramnios, then premature labor will occur. Stretching of the uterine wall is probably the cause of the higher incidence of prematurity in twin and triplet pregnancies.

Physicians now believe that up to thirty percent of premature births are due to infection. Bacteria and other microbes produce toxins that stimulate the defence cells in the body, the white blood cells, of which there are several types. One type, the macrophage, hurries to the site of infection and secretes chemicals that stimulate the immune system in an attempt to restrict the spread of the microbes and kill them off. These chemicals produced by the macrophage have wide-ranging effects. One effect is to stimulate prostaglandin production. As we have seen, prostaglandins can stimulate the muscle of the uterus to contract and also cause the cervix to dilate. It is not surprising, therefore, that if the infection is not treated or overcome by the defence systems of the body it will increase the risk of premature birth.

Infection of a pregnant women's reproductive tract is more likely to occur if nutritional state of the mother is poor and if her general level of health is depressed. Anemia, high blood pressure, poor diet, inadequate prenatal care, together or separately, increase the risk of an infection taking hold. More emphasis must be placed on the proper provision of care for every pregnant mother and every baby during life before birth. Society has an inescapable duty to take care of the next generation. Research must be undertaken to find the mechanisms that cause prematurity. We need only look at the costs of maintaining severely affected premature babies for the whole of their lives to justify the cost of research. The cost can exceed two hundred fifty thousand dollars a year for one such baby. Resources are finite and we need to spend them in the most cost-effective fashion. Prevention is better than cure for the child and family: it is also cheaper.

Several epidemiological studies have shown that maternal lifestyle will affect the incidence of prematurity. Dr. Emile Papiernik and his colleagues in France have undertaken several studies that demonstrate the beneficial effects of modifying adverse factors in the mother's environment. Their studies show that several stressors in the maternal environment and lifestyle increase the risk of prematurity. Even the stress of changing address during pregnancy was associated with an increased risk of premature birth. We have seen how the stress-related hormones from the maternal and fetal adrenal glands provide the precursors from which the placenta produces estrogens. It is, therefore, not surprising that a wide variety of stressors can precipitate the hormone changes that normally lead to increased contraction of the uterine muscle. Many studies have shown that stress can increase the amount of uterine activity and switch contractures to contractions.

Not all prematurity is disastrous. Some premature babies adapt extremely well to an early arrival into the world. As mentioned before Isaac Newton was so small when he was born that it was said that he could have been fitted into a pint pot. Seemingly, it is a paradox that growth-retarded premature babies—that is, babies who are even smaller than they should be at their particular fetal age—often fare better after birth than other babies of the same fetal age. The reason for this is easy to understand. The growth-retarded baby has almost certainly been short of nutrients and oxygen for an appreciable length of time in the uterus. He has responded appropriately and effectively to these adverse conditions by increasing his secretion of cortisol and other stress-related hormones, as well as mobilizing his nutritional reserves. He is a seasoned fighter against adversity. As a result his lungs are likely to be more mature than those of a baby who was unstressed in the uterus and then due to some emergency was suddenly delivered. Indeed the chronically stressed growth-retarded baby may well have made the decision for himself that he is better out than in.

In the early 1950s Dr. Virginia Apgar designed a numerical scale for evaluation of the level of maturation of the newborn baby. The Apgar scale reports on five features that can be expressed as an acronym: Appearance of the newborn baby; Pulse rate; Grimace and facial activity; Activity of the limbs; and Respiration. Each of the five factors is given a score of 0 (lowest), 1, or 2 (highest). The perfect baby score is ten: a perfect ten. These features of the baby's function tell the physician how well the baby's brain is regulating his heart (P) and breathing (R), and the brain's control over muscles of the face (G) and limbs (A). The neonatologist scores the baby at one and five minutes after birth. A healthy baby will have an Apgar score of 7 to 10 at one minute after birth. If the score is lower than 7, the neonatologist may need to provide oxygen to the baby's lungs using a ventilator, to ease the transition from dependence on the placenta to breathing for himself. The baby is gently dried off to lessen the rate at which heat is lost from the body, a process that can be assisted by a radiant warmer. We know that it is very important that the baby be kept warm and maintain his body temperature.

When the Apgar score is less than 3, the neonatologist has much more to do. The first step in resuscitation of a baby who is taking a while to respond to his new environment is to give the oxygen that is no longer arriving from the placenta. Oxygen delivered by a face mask, or a tube in the trachea if necessary, will provide air to the baby until he breathes adequately for himself. In extreme cases the baby may not yet be able to expand his own lungs and breathe by himself, and it may be necessary to provide mechanical ventilation for his immature lungs. We have seen that the fetus lived at an oxygen level about one fifth of that in the outside world. If the newborn baby is over-ventilated, there is a danger of oxygen toxicity that can permanently damage the eyes and lungs. This may seem a catch-22 situation. Too little oxygen and the risk of brain damage increases; but too much oxygen, and damage may occur to the eyes and lungs. If the newborn retina is exposed to high oxygen levels connective tissue fibers grow in among the light-sensitive cells causing blindness. The amount of oxygen delivered to a newborn baby by face mask or other route is carefully regulated by the neonatologist according to various carefully determined procedures based on detailed research findings. These procedures used in the neonatal intensive care unit are the clinical expression of the knowledge that has been gained over the last thirty years in the research laboratory. Thousands of premature babies are alive and healthy today because of the knowledge that has been garnered about how the fetus grows and develops during life before birth.

The long-term outlook for the baby depends on just how prematurely birth actually occurs, the degree of maturation of the fetus at the time, and the level of neonatal care that is available immediately. The major risks of prematurity are brain damage due to hemorrhage, immature development of the stomach and digestive system requiring special feeding regimens, inability to control water and salt concentrations in the body due to immaturity of the kidneys, inadequate lung development requiring assisted ventilation, inability to control heat loss from the body with a consequent loss of body temperature, lack of glucose and calcium that would normally come from the mother across the placenta, and jaundice because the newborn baby's liver is not yet able to get rid of the colored pigments that are produced as the red blood cells break down (bilirubin). The newborn baby is also more susceptible to infection and the effects of stress produced by various stressors. Each of these abnormalities has potential long-term dangers. For example, if the products of red cell pigment breakdown accumulate in the baby's blood they can be deposited in selected parts of the brain, where they produce permanent damage resulting in a variety of neurological problems. Hemorrhage in the brain of the newborn baby can lead to neurological disorders and intellectual deficits. Intracranial hemorrhage (bleeding into the brain) occurs in seventy-five percent of babies under one thousand grams. However, the developing nervous system is remarkably resilient. Even as adults we do not use the whole capacity of our brains. Following even the trauma of a large stroke an adult can re-learn old functions using other parts of the brain. Newborn babies are even more adept at compensating for damage.

The NICU has done its best to mimic the situation inside the uterus. In the past the NICU was always a place in which there was turmoil twenty-four hours a day with high-technology medicine being employed in a dramatic rescue mission to keep very sick babies alive. Some of this drama cannot be avoided because life-threatening situations do often develop dramatically. The sound of beeping monitors and bright lights are all-pervasive. This environment is nothing like the warm, comfortable, reassuring fluid-filled cushioning of the uterus, with very little light and the regular influence of several of the mother's twenty-four-hour rhythms. There are no contractures in the NICU to gently stimulate the newborn baby and modify the sensory input going to his brain. Many NICUs are now conducting small trials of environments that try to simulate the intrauterine situation. This is a sensible attempt to apply what we are learning from research studies to the care of the developing premature baby, especially to his brain. Of course it is work that is highly sensitive and conducted in a very emotional area of medical science. The neonatologist has a difficult path to tread between not doing all he can and doing more than is justified by the current state of knowledge.

The treatment of very premature babies is indeed a modern technological miracle for those babies who survive apparently with no major abnormalities. The problem is that we have no way of determining which babies will have little or no deficit and those that will have long-term handicap of various sorts. The handicap, along with being a personal challenge and misfortune, constitutes a great burden to society. The babies needing the greatest amount of care and attention are not surprisingly the worst affected and hence the ones with the worst prospects.

It is only now being recognized that the follow-up of many brain-damaged babies needs to be for their lifetime. Although there may be little deficit at two years of age, problems may arise later. Pilot studies show that just as catch-up growth may occur in the physical structure of the body, early intervention with educational and other therapies that help the development of the nervous system may be of considerable use. We need to know more about the plasticity of the newborn nervous system. There may be great economic savings in terms of less need for special education if we get these premature babies into programs that address their needs.

Anyone with personal experience of the effects of brain damage will readily recognize what a distressing phenomenon it is. It imposes a lifetime of servitude on the parent to the needs of their offspring; it compels society to make complex and costly provision for care; it diverts medical energy away from other more curable conditions. Most of all it creates human beings unable to fulfill their full potential or make their complete contribution to the community. As a result of perinatal research in the last thirty years in laboratories around the world we are on the brink of enormous leaps of knowledge that could go far to reducing or even eliminating the scourge of prematurity from our society, and thereby dramatically reducing the incidence of brain damage.

Chapter 16

THE FUTURE

What a piece of work is man.

William Shakespeare, *Hamlet*

It was once said that the moral test of government is how that government treats those who are in the dawn of life, the children; those who are in the twilight of life, the elderly; and those who are in the shadows of life—the sick, the needy, and the handicapped.

Dedication of the Hubert H. Humphrey Building, New York, on November 1, 1977. *Congressional Record,* November 4, 1977, Vol. 123, p. 37287.

For each newborn child the future holds out a wealth of unexplored and unrealized promise. Each child is a new book with most of the pages blank. The parental instinct drives us to nurture our children to the utmost of our ability, to give them every chance to reach whatever goals and happiness that are best fitted to their needs and personality. This instinct of parental love is the very strongest human emotion. This love is a deep-seated drive that outshines all other altruism. It exerts itself so strongly that one feels the emotion must have a physical basis; that it must be replicated somewhere in our genes. The love of children is enshrined in art, music, literature, and poetry. Children are the keepers of the future. The torch of life is passed from one generation to the next for the young to seize and carry. The fabric of society is passed along the human chain for each succeeding generation to modify and reconstruct. As we have seen, the ability of each newborn child to carry this lamp, to shape the fabric, initially depends on how well he or she has been nurtured and allowed to develop abilities during life before birth.

Each generation has a sublime and transcendent duty to do everything it can to improve the potential for a better life in the next. I will not address here the vitally important issue of the costs of health care during pregnancy and its relative value when compared with the other demands for expenditure that are placed before society—roads, schools, defense, pensions. However, I would like to focus attention on the need for prevention of those problems that may diminish the quality of life of each newborn baby. It has been shown over and over again that prevention is cheaper and more efficient than cure. Society knows this self-evident fact only too well, yet we still cut back on prenatal care in those disadvantaged sections of the community that would most benefit.

I wish to accentuate the positive, rather than dwell on negatives. We need to think about the needs of children before they are born and make every effort to ensure that they are as healthy as possible when they make that first marvelous cry, "I am here." We need to ensure that pregnant women and their families are well nourished and free from unnecessary stress. We must do everything within our power to reverse the trends of the last twenty years in which the general level of prenatal care has diminished. Experts like Dr. Berry Brazelton have said that no generation of children has been born less well nourished and less well prepared for life after birth than the babies being born today. In a society as endowed with material benefits and knowledge as ours there is a deep shame in this state of affairs. Perhaps it is because newborn infants do not vote that the politicians ignore them.

It is the aim of this book to help any interested parties— students, parents-to-be, politicians, or medical administrators—to understand the process of development through which each fetus must go. We should all marvel at the intricacy of fetal development. Understanding this miraculous process can only induce respect, and out of that respect perhaps will grow a more thoughtful and caring provision for life before birth. Knowledge of fetal development can help us prepare the baby for life after birth. A baby is a very accomplished individual even before birth. He or she has undertaken great feats of growth and development. His brain is already taking in information and deciding how to respond. He has monitored the development of his lungs and heart and decided that he is ready to come and join us in the outside world. The least we can do for him is to give him every opportunity to exploit his capacity.

We stand upon the threshold of knowledge that can truly help improve the lives of many children of the generations to come who would otherwise suffer permanently from the consequences of troubles experienced during life before birth. The unparalleled explosion in research support from the national governments of the industrialized countries over the last fifty years has been gloriously successful. Too successful for some economists—as expectations have often risen faster than they can be fulfilled because of the high cost of medical technology. The sciences of chemistry and physics have unlocked the most intimate secrets of molecular structure so that we can synthesize designer molecules whose structures act as specific keys to specific locks. Such drugs can help prevent seizures, dramatically shorten the duration and consequences of infection, treat diabetes, and lower maternal blood pressure. Technological advances have produced instrumentation for diagnosis and treatment that only the most affluent can afford. In perinatal medicine the ability to monitor very small premature babies until they can live an independent life has depended heavily on the development of electronic monitors and computer-based recorders. A veritable arsenal of pharmacological agents and solutions has been prepared by pharmaceutical companies as a result of basic animal research. For example, as a result of research based on lung function in fetal and premature animals we now have artificial surfactants to help open the air sacs of the premature baby.

There is a long way to go scientifically, ethically, and politically before many tricky personal and social problems are solved. We flounder in the face of such decisions as when to turn off life support for babies in the NICU. Similar problems are faced with adult patients. We grope for answers to the ethics of termination of unwanted pregnancies rather than bring children into a world where they are not wanted immediately. We avoid the philosophical debate of the differences between abortion and birth control; both prevent a specific and unique genotype from coming into existence.

The study of disease processes has greatly increased life-expectancy over the last century. It has also improved the quality of life. A good example of this is the polio vaccine. I can remember as a Boy Scout at camp in 1952 being forbidden to swim in the local river. The sun was brilliant, the high cliffs of Derbyshire rose above our campsite, and the water glistened, but we were not allowed to swim. Why? Polio was like the AIDS virus of today. The polio virus is spread by water, entering the body and settling down in the nerve cells of the brain and spinal cord that control voluntary muscles. It destroys these critical cells so that the muscles they supply cannot be used. Once the nerve cells are destroyed the muscles they serve are permanently paralysed. One member of my scout patrol contracted polio. In a way he was lucky, because the virus had attacked only a small part of his spinal cord and his right arm was only partially affected. To outside appearances his arm was not affected but it was sufficiently weak that he could not lift an axe. Unable to do this, he could not qualify for the back-woodsman badge. The other scouts jeered him as he tried to cut down the tree he needed to fell to pass the test. He wasn't adequately crippled to evoke sympathy—just enough to provoke this extraordinary cruelty of children. Fortunately a generous scout master passed him all the same. Many of my generation have stories to tell like this about the terrible toll of polio.

Polio was conquered by the production of a vaccine grown on monkey kidneys. We forget so quickly. I often ask those who are against research in general, and research using animals in particular, what they know about polio. I can date their age by the facial response. If they are younger than thirty years all they remember is that they have had a vaccination. Thanks to the recently developed vaccine, the iron lungs used before the vaccine was developed are no longer needed. They are stacked away, forgotten, lined up along the walls of storerooms like so many disused and obsolete automobiles. Unfortunately, unlike polio there are many equally damaging conditions that arise before or shortly after birth that have not yet been conquered. The goals of perinatal research *must* be to prevent cerebral palsy, to improve our understanding of prematurity, to give every baby its right to a sound body and mind when she or he is born, and perhaps one day make the NICU as obsolete as the iron lung.

Modern biomedical science stands on the threshold of many critical advances that will help both the fetus and the newborn baby. Already pediatric surgeons are attempting to repair life-threatening abnormalities while the fetus is still in the uterus. At present, the success rate for such surgeries is unacceptably low. The problems that stand in the way of further advances are not surgical problems. Researchers who study the activity of the uterine muscle during pregnancy know that most forms of stress lead to increased contractile activity of the uterus. Thus it is not surprising that the consequence of surgery on the fetus in the uterus is too often the premature delivery of a baby who is not yet ready to leave the uterus. We need more information on the factors that control the contractile activity of the uterine muscle. The ability to control the contractility of uterine muscle will be necessary before regular success will be achieved by the pioneer surgeons who are trying to develop intrauterine surgical procedures for fetuses with life-threatening defects. Drugs that will control the activity of the uterine muscle are even more necessary for efficient management of premature labor.

We need to know more about the effects of abnormal sleep/wakefulness patterns in the fetus, the premature and the full-term baby. The ultrasound shows us that each fetus has his or her own personality in late pregnancy. We need to know how abnormalities of prenatal development can lead to SIDS, to brain damage, to heart defects, and all the long-term disabilities such as autism and other behavioral problems from which so many children suffer. We need more information if we are to help our children and our grandchildren to triumph over the many challenges that will beset them in the years to come: global warming, environmental pollution, racial and religious harmony. These are problems for bright minds and well-adjusted people to solve.

I believe there is valid hope that we can understand the causes of such conditions as high maternal blood pressure in pregnancy that lead to fetal growth retardation and brain retardation. The tools that biomedical science has put at our disposal are miraculous. We can use the ultrasound as a video camera on the developing fetus. We can track the fetus' heart beat and can follow his responses to sound and uterine contractures.

However, there is much to learn. We need more research to understand why the placenta may not be able to keep up with the fetus' needs in some conditions. If the placenta is inadequate can we devise ways to feed the baby, by the amniotic cavity for example? What is necessary now are firm data on the advantages and risks, so that we can decide whether there might be situations where it may be advantageous to prolong pregnancy and to keep the fetuses in the uterus a little longer to allow them to mature. We have seen that the sleep patterns of full-term babies born at forty weeks of pregnancy are different from those of babies born prematurely and reared in an NICU until the time at which they should have been born. Development outside the uterus may not be as advantageous as development inside the uterus at critical phases of the baby's program.

Abnormal inputs to the fetal brain during fetal life may alter the correct amount and sequence of fetal brain development. We have seen how dietary problems in early and late gestation have different effects on appetite and weight control throughout life. We do not know how diet and the intrauterine environment combine to produce changes in the brain that may have permanent effects. Normal function in our complex twentieth, soon to be twenty-first, century requires the correct interaction of our senses, our nervous systems to control the activities that produce the feedback from our senses and the central controlling computer. Trouble in any one of these components leading to an imbalance of the system may result in a child not reaching his full potential.

Creativity will be the key to life in the twenty-first century. We do not know the fundamental causes of creativity but we do know that damaged brains and stunted bodies are not optimally creative. The dividend from more research investment in terms of avoiding the problems and improving the quality of fetal life will be enormous for society.

Everyone is entitled to a dream, a vision of how they would like the future to be. The long-term resolution of all types of problems—personal, financial, and social—is best achieved by discovering the root cause and removing it. Researchers have been known to say that behind each problem lurks a smaller problem that is easier to solve and indeed must be solved first, before the big problem can be addressed. Sir James Black, the Nobel Laureate who was responsible for the discovery of the most effective treatments for some major heart conditions and stomach ulcers, told me on a visit to my laboratory that he had been advised as a young scientist to divide each problem into its smaller components. We should keep doing this until it is no longer possible to divide it. Then the real problem will surface.

Advice for the laboratory is not always translatable to our everyday life. However, I hope this book has given the reader enough insight into life before birth to see that much remains to be done to improve the chances of every newborn baby as they enter the world. Our vision of the future must include a society that pays attention to prenatal care and nutrition; a society that is orientated to the young. The young are the future, even though as politicians point out children do not vote. If we care enough about the health and happiness of our children and our children's children, we will be prepared to pay the necessary price for the research and social services that will reduce the incidence of prematurity and its attendant long-term handicap, and decrease the incidence of growth retardation and provide every child with the maximum opportunity to fulfill his full potential.

The 1990s have been called the Decade of the Brain. I would like to see the first century of the next millennium called the Century of the Child. If we have the resolve, the research tools are in place. We also have the knowledge of what we do not know, an essential prerequisite to progress. It is important to know the extent of one's ignorance before starting out on any endeavor. All society needs is the commitment and the will.

The marvels of life before birth are worth pondering. Whether one believes that the program that drives our development in the uterus is the result of immutable physical and chemical laws or that it expresses the divine concern of a benign spiritual power there is little doubt that "we are fearfully and wonderfully made." I look forward to a time when adequate maternal care will be available to all mothers (and fathers) who have made the decision to make their ultimate contribution to the continuation of life on our planet; to a time when the care of the fetus in the uterus is as much a matter of concern as the care of a juvenile diabetic, a middle-aged coronary care patient; or a beloved grandparent; to a time when Life Before Birth is understood and cherished for all its wonder; to a time when each newborn baby not only cries *"I am here"* but cries *"I am perfectly made."*

GLOSSARY

ACTH See adrenocorticotropin.

Acromegaly Disease in which there is excessive secretion of growth hormone.

Adaptation The decrease in the nervous response to a stimulus that is maintained constant.

Adhesion molecules Specialized molecules that stick cells together helping tissues to form their unique and individual shape.

Adrenaline Hormone secreted by the cells at the center of the adrenal gland in response to stressful situations.

Adrenocorticotropin (ACTH) Hormone produced by the pituitary that controls the secretion of cortisol by the adrenal cortex.

Afferent nervous system The nerve fibers which carry information to the brain and spinal cord.

Air sac Bubble of air at the end of the air passages. The cells lining the air sac are so thin that oxygen easily diffuses into the blood.

Aldosterone Hormone which controls salt composition of the body, secreted by the outer cells of the adrenal gland.

Amino acids Small molecules that are the building blocks from which proteins are constructed.

Amniotic cavity The protective sac that forms around the developing embryo; both ends of the embryo's digestive system open into the amniotic cavity.

Amniotic fluid Fluid in the amniotic cavity made up of fetal urine and secretions from the lungs and digestive system.

Amnion Fetal membrane around the amniotic cavity.

Anemia Shortage of hemoglobin in the red blood cells.

Antidiuretic hormone Hormone produced by the pituitary gland in response to stressful conditions, especially at times of water shortage when it instructs the kidney to retain water.

Aorta The largest artery in the body, carrying blood from the left ventricle to the head, chest, abdomen, and limbs.

Apgar score A scale to assess the well-being of the newborn baby; it evaluates activity of the limbs, pulse, appearance of the face, facial movements, and breathing.

Asymmetrical growth retardation The uneven growth retardation that occurs late in fetal life. In times of shortage of oxygen or nutrients the fetus protects his brain and structures close to the head. Growth retardation is less likely to occur in the brain than in other structures, such as liver, legs and trunk.

Atom The smallest complete portion of any chemical element.

Atrium, pl. atria The two, thinner-walled, smaller cavities in the heart. The right atrium receives the blood returning to the heart from the body and the left atrium receives the blood returning to the heart from the lungs.

Auditory cortex The part of the cerebral cortex of the brain that processes sound information.

Autonomic nervous system The part of the nervous system that carries messages to control the function of glands, the heart and the muscle cells that control the amount of blood that flows through the arteries. These nerves cannot be controlled voluntarily.

Axon The main outgrowth from a nerve cell that carries information to other cells, often over great distances (see dendrite).

Blastocyst The stage of embryonic development after fertilization, when the developing zygote divides many times to form a small cluster of cells with a central cavity.

Brainstem The part of the brain nearest the spinal cord which contains the nerve cells that control the basic body functions such as breathing and the action of the heart.

Cardiovascular system The heart and blood vessels.

Catecholamines Group of hormones that includes adrenaline and noradrenaline produced by the adrenal gland and the autonomic nervous system.

Cell cycle The regular progression of growth and synthesis of new DNA and cell division.

Cell differentiation Specialization of cells to perform specific tasks. Normally cells stop dividing after they have differentiated.

Central nervous system The brain and spinal cord.

Cerebral cortex The most highly developed parts of the brain responsible for detailed processing of sensory information, as well as complex functions such as judgement and reasoning.

Cerebrospinal fluid A protective fluid produced deep within the brain which flows out to surround the brain and spinal cord (see ventricle).

Cervix The tight fibrous tissue at the outlet from the uterus to the vagina.

Chimera Organism produced by the fusion of cells from two embryos so early in development that only one organism forms. A chimera is made up of a mosaic of cells derived from the two embryos.

Chorionic gonadotrophin Hormone produced by the trophoblast that acts as a signal from the fetus to the mother's ovary to continue the life of the corpus luteum.

Chromosomes Long thread-like structures within the nucleus of the cell on which the genes are strung.

Chronobiology Study of the influence of time on biological events and systems.

Circadian rhythm Rhythm within the suprachiasmatic nucleus that lasts approximately twenty-four hours and is not dependent on outside cues (see entrainment).

Contractions Strong contraction of the muscle of the uterus at the time of birth. Contractions usually last only a minute, eventually occurring every two to three minutes (see contractures).

Contractures Episodes of contraction of the uterine muscle that occur about once an hour, last three to fifteen minutes, and cause only a small increase in the pressure in the uterus. Contractures occur throughout pregnancy (see contractions).

Corpus luteum Formed by the follicle after the ovum has been released at the time of ovulation. The corpus luteum produces progesterone, a hormone that plays a key role in the maintenance of the pregnancy.

Cortex Name given to the outer zone of a structure that can be clearly divided into inner and outer areas, such as the cerebral cortex and the adrenal cortex.

Corticotropin releasing hormone (CRH) Hormone produced by the hypothalamus that regulates the production of ACTH by the pituitary gland.

Cortisol Hormone produced by outer layers of the adrenal cortex.

CRH See corticotropin releasing hormone.

Cyclic AMP Intracellular regulator molecule released within a cell when hormones and other cell function regulators act on the cell to alter its activity.

Cytoplasm Fluid which is contained within the plasma membrane of the cell but outside the nucleus.

Dehydroepiandrosterone sulfate (DHEAS) Hormone produced by the adrenal gland in both the mother and fetus that is converted to estrogen by the placenta.

Dendrites Small tentacle-like outgrowths from nerve cells by which they make contact with other nerve cells nearby (see axon).

Deoxyribonucleic acid (DNA) Chain-like structure of repeating units. The sequence of the units carries the genetic code from which complex molecules are synthesized.

DHEAS See dehydroepiandrosterone sulfate.

Diffusion Passive process whereby substances in solution move from an area of high concentration to one of low concentration.

Digestive system Develops from the embryonic gut, forming the feeding tract from the mouth to the anus.

DNA See deoxyribonucleic acid.

Dominant follicle The one of several follicles produced in each ovarian cycle in women that matures faster than all the others. This is the follicle that will be ovulated during that cycle.

Dorsal horn Entry point of sensory pathways into the spinal cord.

Ductus arteriosus A very short blood vessel that connects the pulmonary artery to the aorta in the fetus. During fetal life blood passes from the pulmonary artery to the aorta, bypassing the lungs which are not yet functional. The ductus arteriosus closes after birth.

Ectoderm The outermost layer of the three sheets of cells that make up the early embryo in the third week after fertilization of the egg by the sperm.

Ectopic pregnancy The development of the embryo outside the body of the uterus. The most common site is the Fallopian tube.

Ectopic pregnancies do not usually form an adequate placenta and, therefore, generally die within the first few weeks after they are formed. They rarely develop to the point where the fetus could survive by itself.

Efferent nervous system The nerve fibers that carry information away from the brain and spinal cord.

Electromyography Method by which small electrodes are used to record electrical activity of muscles as they contract.

Embryonic gut The primitive digestive tract.

Endocrine gland Specialized cell groups producing instructional molecules called hormones.

Endoderm The innermost layer of the three sheets of cells that make up the early embryo in the third week after fertilization of the egg by the sperm.

Enzymes Specialized proteins within the cell that regulates the speed at which critical chemical reactions take place.

Entrainment Conversion of a circadian rhythm into one that is fixed to an outside rhythm such as the day/night or light/dark cycle.

Epidemiology The science that deals with statistical relationships between environmental situations and disease.

Epithelium Layer of cells that lines a surface.

Estrogens Steroid hormone produced by the ovary, especially at the time of ovulation. Estrogens are also produced by the placenta, and play a major role in stimulating the uterine muscle to contract in labor and delivery.

Facilitated diffusion The form of diffusion that utilizes a carrier to speed up the process.

Fallopian tube The narrow tube that begins near the ovary and conducts the ovum to its implantation site in the uterus.

Fetal Alcohol Syndrome Impaired development of the fetus, especially the brain, as a result of chronic exposure to alcohol consumed by the mother.

Fetal membranes The sheets of cells that surround the fluid in the amniotic cavity and lie next to the lining of the uterus. They are formed from the trophoblast.

Follicle The dense grouping of cells around the developing ovum. Each follicle has a single ovum at its center. Each month usually only one follicle becomes dominant and ovulates.

Foramen ovale Hole in the septum between the right and left atrium. Well oxygenated blood from the placenta passes through the foramen ovale and goes straight to the fetal brain.

Forebrain Front part of the developing brain that becomes the cerebral cortex and the hypothalamus.

Gametes Specialized sex cells, the ova in the female and the spermatozoa in the male. Each gamete has half the number of chromosomes of the other cells of the body.

Genes The molecular structures that carry the codes for producing the complex molecules that make up the cells of the body. Genes are the blueprints for the developing fetus. It is thought that there are 100,000 genes in each human cell.

Genome The total of all the genetic factors in the chromosomes.

Glial cells Cells in the nervous system that lie between the nerve cells and their dendrites and axons. Glial cells have important nutritive and insulating functions.

Glucose The body's main source of energy.

Glucose transporter Specialized molecule that speeds the rate at which glucose is transported across the placenta and other membranes (see facilitated diffusion).

Glycogen Storage form of glucose, made up of long chains of glucose molecules.

Gonad The glands responsible for producing the sex hormones and the gametes; the testis in the male, the ovary in the female.

Grey matter Areas of the central nervous system that contain the nerve cells and are grey in color.

Growth factors Paracrine and endocrine regulator compounds that alter the rate of growth of different cell types.

Growth hormone Hormone produced by the pituitary gland. It plays a major role in the control of growth, especially after birth.

Growth retardation Slowing of fetal growth from its normal rate. If the growth retardation occurs early in pregnancy it produces symmetrical growth retardation. If it occurs late it produces asymmetrical growth retardation.

Habituation The decrease in the nervous response to a stimulus that is constantly maintained.

Hemoglobin Specialized molecule in the red blood cells that collects oxygen and carbon dioxide molecules and carries them around the body.

Hindbrain Part of the developing brain that will form the centers that control the most basic activities of the body, such as the cardiovascular system and breathing.

Hormone A chemical messenger, produced by an endocrine gland, which passes into the bloodstream and circulates around the body to give instructions to other cells that have a specific receptor for the hormone.

Horn Part of the spinal cord that contains a dense grouping of nerve cells.

Hypoglycemia A shortage of glucose in the blood.

Hypoxemia Situation in which there is insufficient oxygen in the blood.

Hypoxia Shortage of oxygen in cells.

Hypothalamus Part of the forebrain containing the nerve cells that control production of many hormones.

Hypothyroidism Insufficient thyroxine in the blood.

Immune system The defense mechanisms of the body that fight off infections.

Inferior vena cava The large vein in the abdomen that carries blood back to the heart.

Inner cell mass The group of cells in the early embryo that lie beneath the trophoblast and will form the fetus.

Intestine Narrow part of the digestive tract which leads from the stomach to the anus.

Involuntary muscles Muscle cells such as those in blood vessels and the uterus that cannot be consciously controlled.

Ion Electrically charged form in which most atoms exist in solution.

Lactic acid A product of the breakdown of glucose under conditions of oxygen shortage.

Laryngo-tracheal diverticulum Pouch that grows out from the front end of the embryonic gut to form the lungs.

Larynx Upper portion of the airway to the lungs; contains the vocal cords.

Lateral horn Collection of nerve cells in the spinal cord that control the automatic functions of glands and involuntary muscles.

Lipids A collective name for all fats.

Macrophage One of the cells of the immune system. Some macrophages circulate in the blood; others are positioned in the tissues to respond rapidly to foreign agents.

Mammals Group of higher animals, including man, distinguished by the fact that the young develop within the mother and the mother feeds the newborn with milk from the breast.

Matrix The collection of supporting compounds that make up the fluid between cells.

Meconium Thick greenish contents of the fetal digestive tract, made up of dead cells and old secretions. Meconium may pass into the amniotic fluid if the fetus is stressed.

Medulla Name given to the inner zone of a structure that can be clearly divided into inner and outer areas.

Menstruation Monthly shedding of the lining of the uterus, occurring when fertilization has not taken place. The uterine lining is prepared for implantation of an embryo, but will not always be needed.

Mesoderm The middle layer of the three sheets of cells that make up the early embryo in the third week after fertilization of the egg by the sperm.

Miscarriage Loss of the embryo within the first few weeks of pregnancy.

Morula The solid cluster of cells formed from the fertilized ovum as it divides while passing down the Fallopian tube.

Myoglobin Large molecule in the muscle cell that collects the oxygen muscle cells use to produce energy when they contract.

Myometrium The muscle cells of the uterus.

Neonatal intensive care unit (NICU) Hospital unit that provides specialized support for the premature baby.

Neonatology Branch of pediatric medicine which deals with newborn babies.

Nerve growth factor A growth factor produced by some tissues that stimulates the growth of nerve fibers, particularly sensory nerve fibers.

Nervous system The body's main control system comprised of the afferent nervous system, which obtains the information on the world outside and inside the body; the central nervous system (the brain and spinal cord), which processes the information; and the efferent nervous system, which sends out orders to the muscles and glands to respond to the information received.

Neural tube Midline column of cells that runs the full length of the embryo at the fourth week of life and will become the central nervous system.

Noradrenaline Both a hormone and a transmitter produced by the adrenal gland and the nervous system; it plays an important role in the body's response to stressful situations.

Notochord A midline column of cells that appears in the embryo at the end of the second week of embryonic life and organizes the formation of the spinal cord.

Nucleus Has two meanings; 1) the command center of each cell in which the chromosomes are located; 2) collections of nerve cells in the brain that control a particular function.

Optic nerve Nerve connecting the eye to the brain.

Optic vesicle Cup that grows out from the brain and will become the eye.

Organ Major structures of the body, made up of several different types of cells (see tissues).

Ovary Female sex gland in which the ova and female sex hormones are produced.

Ovulation The release of a mature ovum from the ovary. In women ovulation occurs approximately once a month. The ovum, or egg, is swept away from the surface of the ovary and into the Fallopian tube down which it passes into the uterus.

Ovum (pl. ova) The ovum grows slowly in the middle of a specialized structure called the follicle within the ovary. The cells of the follicle provide nourishment for the ovum. At any one time there are several ova in the ovary at various stages of development. In women, just before ovulation, one ovum begins to mature faster than the rest. It is this ovum which is ovulated. Occasionally more than one ovum is ovulated and multiple fetuses may be produced.

Oxygen dissociation curve Relationship between the partial pressure of oxygen in the blood and the amount of oxygen carried by hemoglobin.

Oxytocin Hormone released from nerve cells that are in the mother's hypothalamus. Oxytocin stimulates the uterine muscle to contract.

Paracrine regulator A molecule that carries information from one cell to another in its neighborhood without passing into the blood stream.

Paradoxical response to oxygen lack The fetus responds to lack of oxygen by making fewer breathing movements. In contrast the newborn breathes more actively when oxygen is short.

Paraventricular nucleus Collection of nerve cells in the hypothalamus that secretes several hormones including CRH, the hormone that controls the secretion of ACTH.

Partial pressure The proportion of the overall pressure in the atmosphere contributed by each gas.

Peripheral nervous system Nerves leading into and out of the brain and spinal cord.

Pharynx The junction of the mouth, back of the nose, and the larynx.

Pituitary gland Master endocrine gland that lies beneath the hypothalamus, and secretes at least eight hormones, including ACTH.

Placenta The organ of exchange of gases and nutrients between the mother and fetus. It is formed from both maternal and fetal cells.

Placental lactogen Hormone produced by the fetal layers of the placenta that acts both on the fetus and the mother to produce growth and to prepare the mother's breasts to produce milk.

Plasma membrane Envelope around the cell that regulates the passage of molecules in and out of the cell.

Platelets Disc-shaped structures that circulate in the blood and collect to form blood clots in wounds.

Platelet derived growth factor Growth promoting molecule produced by the platelets in the blood.

Polyhydramnios A condition in which there is an excess of amniotic fluid in the amniotic cavity around the fetus.

Progesterone A steroid hormone produced by the ovary during the second half of the ovarian cycle, known as the luteal phase of the cycle. Progesterone is also produced by the placenta. Progesterone plays a major role in quieting the contractions of the uterus and maintaining pregnancy.

Prostaglandins Produced from lipids, prostaglandins are complex molecules that act as both endocrine and paracrine regulators.

Pulmonary artery Artery that takes blood from the right ventricle to the lungs. The blood in the pulmonary artery is poorly oxygenated and in the newborn will pick up oxygen from the lungs.

Pulmonary circulation The blood supply to and from the lungs, as distinguished from the systemic circulation which serves the body as a whole.

Pulmonary veins Veins that lead the blood back from the lungs to the left atrium. Blood in these veins is well oxygenated as oxygen has just been picked up from the lungs.

Rapid eye movement (REM) sleep The period of sleep during which there are rapid movements of the eyes and movement of body muscles is inhibited. It is during this period of sleep when dreaming occurs in adults.

Receptor A specialized molecule on the membrane or in the nucleus of the cell to which signalling messengers bind. As a result of the binding of the messenger and the receptor, key mechanisms in the cell are either activated or inhibited.

REM See rapid eye movement.

Respiratory center Collection of nerve cells in the hindbrain that regulate the activity of the breathing muscles.

Ribonucleic acid (RNA) Coding chain produced from DNA that carries the genetic blueprint from the nucleus out to the cytoplasm.

RNA See ribonucleic acid.

Septum Partition that divides one cavity or structure from another. In the heart the inter-atrial septum divides the right atrium from the left, and the inter-ventricular septum separates the right ventricle from the left ventricle.

Sex chromosomes The pair of chromosomes that differs between males and females. In females there are two x-chromosomes; males have one x- and one y-chromosome. The y-chromosome carries the information that provides the signal for the development of male structures throughout the body, including the reproductive organs.

SIDS See Sudden Infant Death Syndrome.

Sperm The specialized male gamete, or sex cell, that fertilizes the ovum to produce the embryo. The scientific form of the name is spermatozoon (pl. spermatozoa).

Stem cell Undifferentiated cell which develops into different cell types.

Stress response The changes in body function in response to a stressful situation.

Stress test Observation of changes in the fetal heart rate when the uterus contracts and oxygen availability to the fetus decreases.

Stressor An unusual situation to which the body must respond to maintain its normal balanced function. A stressor usually produces a stress response.

Sudden Infant Death Syndrome (SIDS) Death of a newborn baby, with no apparent cause even when an autopsy is performed, between one month and one year.

Superior vena cava The large vein that carries blood back to the heart from the head, neck and arms.

Suprachiasmatic nucleus Small group of nerve cells in the hypothalamus having an intrinsic circadian rhythm.

Supraoptic nucleus Collection of nerve cells in the hypothalamus which secrete oxytocin.

Surfactant Combination of fat and protein molecules that line the air sacs in the lungs, lowering the tension in the walls of the sac and allowing it to stay open so that air can go in and out.

Symmetrical growth retardation The type of growth retardation that occurs early in fetal life at the time that cells are dividing. As a result the body will contain fewer cells all over and will be symmetrically growth retarded (see asymmetric growth retardation).

Synapse The junction between two nerve cells.

Systemic circulation The blood supply to and from the general body as distinguished from the pulmonary circulation which serves the lungs.

Teratogen Environmental toxic compound that permanently alters the development of the embryo.

Testis (pl. testes) Male sex gland in which the spermatozoa and male hormones are produced.

Thromboxane An endocrine and paracrine regulator produced by the clotting platelets in the blood.

Thyroxine Hormone produced by the thyroid gland that plays a major role in the body's response to cold temperatures.

Tissue A group of cells of the same type.

Tocodynamometer Pressure-sensitive device that is strapped to the abdomen of the pregnant woman in an attempt to record uterine contraction.

Trachea The main airway from the larynx to the lungs.

Transmitter Chemical messenger that carries information across the gap between cells.

Transposition of the great vessels An abnormality of fetal development in which the aorta and pulmonary artery develop from the wrong chambers of the heart.

Triplet A specific sequence of three blocks in RNA that instructs the protein-producing machinery of the cell to place a particular amino acid next on a protein chain.

Trophoblast The outer wall of the early developing embryo. This layer will make contact with the uterine lining and form the placenta and fetal membranes.

Type I cell Flat irregular-shaped cells that line the air sacs and comprise the barrier between the air and the body fluids.

Type II cell Cells of the air sac lining which produce surfactant.

Umbilical artery The artery in the umbilical cord that carries fetal blood to the placenta, where oxygen is picked up and carbon dioxide and waste products are released from the fetal blood into the mother's blood.

Umbilical cord The connection between the fetus and the placenta which contains the blood vessels that carry blood from the fetus to the placenta and back.

Umbilical vein The vein in the umbilical cord that carries the fetal blood from the placenta to the fetus. The blood in the umbilical vein, rich in oxygen and nutrients obtained from the mother, joins the inferior vena cava in the abdomen.

Ureter Tube leading from the kidney down which urine passes to the bladder.

Ultrasound High frequency sound waves that will bounce off surfaces where the density of tissues differ. They can be used to form a picture of the fetus in the uterus.

Ventral horn Collection of nerve cells that control the muscle cells used for movement (see voluntary muscles).

Ventricle This word is used for two unrelated structures. 1) The thicker walled cavities on the right and left of the heart, and 2) the main cavities in the center of the brain that contain cerebrospinal fluid.

Voluntary muscles Muscle cells used for the body's movements that we can control (see involuntary muscle).

White matter Areas of the central nervous system that contain mostly nerve fibers and few nerve cells and are white in color.

Zygote The first cell of the embryo. It is a single cell formed from the fusion of the sperm and the egg.

INDEX